W9-CKU-554

Histological Typing of Female Genital Tract Tumours

R. E. Scully, T. A. Bonfiglio, R. J. Kurman,
S. G. Silverberg, and E. J. Wilkinson

In Collaboration with Pathologists in 10 Countries

Second Edition

With 200 Figures

Springer-Verlag
Berlin Heidelberg New York
London Paris Tokyo
Hong Kong Barcelona
Budapest

Editorial Committee

R. E. Scully
Chairman, Classification and Nomenclature Committee
International Society of Gynecological Pathologists
Massachusetts General Hospital
32 Fruit Street, Boston, MA 02114, USA

H. E. Poulsen
Head, WHO Collaborating Center for the Histological
Classification of Female Genital Tract Tumours
Herlev Hospital, Ringvej 75, 2730 Herlev, Denmark

L. H. Sobin
Head, WHO Collaborating Center
for the International Histological Classification of Tumours
Armed Forces Institute of Pathology
Alaska and 14th St., Washington, DC 20306-6000, USA

First edition published by WHO in 1975 as No. 13 in the International Histological Classification of Tumours series

ISBN 3-540-57157-4 Springer-Verlag Berlin Heidelberg New York
ISBN 0-387-57157-4 Springer-Verlag New York Berlin Heidelberg

Library of Congress Cataloging-in-Publication Data
Histological typing of female genital tract tumours / R. E. Scully... [et al.] ; in collaboration with pathologists in
10 countries. – 2nd ed. p. cm. – (International histological classification of tumours) Rev. ed. of: Histological
typing of female genital tract tumours / H. E. Poulsen, C. W. Taylor, in collaboration with L. H. Sobin and
pathologists in nine countries. 1975. Includes bibliographical references and index.
ISBN 3-540-57157-4 (alk. paper) – ISBN 0-387-57157-4 (alk. paper)
1. Generative organs, Female – Tumors – Histopathology – Atlases. 2. Generative organs, Female-tumors-Clas-
sification. I. Scully, Robert E. (Robert Edward), 1921– . II. Poulsen, H. E. (Hemming Engelund), 1921– . Histological Typing of female genital tract tumours. III. Series: International histological classification of tumours
(Unnumbered) [DNLM: 1. Genital Neoplasms, Female – pathology – atlases. 2. Genital Neoplasms, Female –
classification – atlases. 3. Genitalia, Female – pathology – atlases. WP 15 H673 1994] RC280.G5H57 1994
616.99'265-dc20 DNLM/DLC for Library of Congress 93-48063 CIP

This work is subject to copyright. All rights are reserved, whether the whole or part of the material is concerned,
specifically the rights of translation, reprinting, reuse of illustrations, recitation, broadcasting, reproduction on
microfilm or in any other way, and storage in data banks. Duplication of this publication or parts thereof is per-
mitted only under the provisions of the German Copyright Law of September 9, 1965, in its current version, and
permission for use must always be obtained from Springer-Verlag. Violations are liable for prosecution under
the German Copyright Law.

© Springer-Verlag Berlin Heidelberg 1994
Printed in Germany

The use of general descriptive names, registered names, trademarks, etc. in this publication does not imply, even
in the absence of a specific statement, that such names are exempt from the relevant protective laws and regula-
tions and therefore free for general use.

Product liability: The publishers cannot guarantee the accuracy of any information about dosage and applica-
tion contained in this book. In every individual case the user must check such information by consulting the relevant literature.

Reproduction of the figures: Gustav Dreher GmbH, Stuttgart
Typesetting and printing: Appl, Wemding. Binding: Schäffer, Grünstadt
25/3111 – 5 4 3 2 1 – Printed on acid-free paper

Participants

Committee on Classification and Nomenclature of the International Society of Gynecological Pathologists

Scully, R. E., Dr., Chairman
Massachusetts General Hospital, Boston, Massachusetts, USA

Subcommittee on Uterine Corpus

Silverberg, S. G., Dr., Chairman
Department of Pathology, George Washington University, Washington, D. C., USA

Dallenbach-Hellweg, G., Dr.
Institut für Pathologie, Mannheim, Germany

Ferenczy, A., Dr.
Departments of Pathology and Obstetrics and Gynaecology, McGill University, Montreal, Canada

Fox, H., Dr.
Department of Pathological Sciences, University of Manchester, Manchester, UK

Gompel, C., Dr.
Department of Pathology, University of Brussels, Brussels, Belgium

Kempson, R. L., Dr.
Laboratory of Surgical Pathology, Stanford University, Stanford, California, USA

Kraus, F. T., Dr.
Department of Pathology, Washington University, St. Louis, Missouri,
USA

Kurman, R. J., Dr.
Departments of Pathology and Gynaecology and Obstetrics,
Johns Hopkins University, Baltimore, Maryland, USA

Miller, A. W., Dr.
Department of Pathology, Good Samaritan Hospital, Downers Grove,
Illinois, USA

Taki, I., Dr.
Department of Obstetrics and Gynaecology, Osaka Police Hospital,
Osaka, Japan

Subcommittee on Gestational Trophoblastic Disease

Kurman, R. J., Dr., Chairman
Departments of Pathology and Gynaecology and Obstetrics,
Johns Hopkins University, Baltimore, Maryland, USA

Driscoll, S. G., Dr.
Department of Pathology, Harvard University, Boston, Massachusetts,
USA

Fox, H., Dr.
Department of Pathological Sciences, University of Manchester,
Manchester, UK

Goldstein, D. P., Dr.
Department of Obstetrics & Gynaecology, Harvard University, Boston,
Massachusetts, USA

Mazur, M. T., Dr.
Department of Pathology, University of Syracuse, Syracuse, New York,
USA

Ober, W. B., Dr. (Deceased)
Department of Pathology, University of Medicine and Dentistry of
New Jersey, Newark, New Jersey, USA

Szulman, A. E., Dr.
Department of Pathology, University of Pittsburgh, Pittsburgh,
Pennsylvania, USA

Twiggs, L. B., Dr.
Department of Obstetrics and Gynaecology, University of Minnesota,
Minneapolis, Minnesota, USA

Yamaguchi, K., Dr.
Department of Pathology, University of Tokyo, Tokyo, Japan

Subcommittee on Uterine Cervix and Vagina

Bonfiglio, T. A., Dr., Chairman
Department of Pathology, University of Rochester, Rochester,
New York, USA

Crum, C. P., Dr.
Department of Pathology, Harvard University, Boston, Massachusetts,
USA

Fu, Y.-S., Dr.
Department of Pathology, University of California, Los Angeles,
California, USA

Kurman, R. J., Dr.
Departments of Pathology and Gynaecology and Obstetrics,
Johns Hopkins University, Baltimore, Maryland, USA

Okagaki, T., Dr.
Departments of Laboratory Medicine, Pathology, and Obstetrics
and Gynaecology, University of Minnesota, Minneapolis, Minnesota,
USA

Prade, M., Dr.
Department of Histopathology, Gustave-Roussy Institute, Villejuif
Cedex, France

Riotton, G., Dr.
Department of Pathology, University of Geneva, Geneva, Switzerland

Russell, P., Dr.
Department of Anatomical Pathology, University of Sydney, Sydney,
Australia

Taki, I., Dr.
Department of Obstetrics and Gynaecology, Osaka Police Hospital,
Osaka, Japan

Vooijs, G. P., Dr.
Department of Pathology, University of Nijmegen, Nijmegen,
The Netherlands

Subcommittee on Vulva

Wilkinson, E. J., Dr., Chairman
Departments of Pathology and Obstetrics and Gynaecology,
University of Florida, Gainesville, Florida, USA

Friedrich, E. G., Dr. (Deceased)
Department of Obstetrics and Gynaecology, University of Florida,
Gainesville, Florida, USA

Fu, Y.-S., Dr.
Department of Pathology, University of California, Los Angeles,
California, USA

Hart, W. R., Dr.
Department of Pathology, Cleveland Clinic Foundation, Cleveland,
Ohio, USA

Kaufman, R. H., Dr.
Departments of Obstetrics and Gynaecology and Pathology,
Baylor University, Houston, Texas, USA

Kraus, F. T., Dr.
Department of Pathology, Washington University, St. Louis, Missouri,
USA

Lynch, R. P., Dr.
Department of Pathology, Health One University Hospital, Fridley,
Minnesota, USA

General Preface to the Series

Among the prerequisites for comparative studies of cancer are international agreement on histological criteria for the definition and classification of cancer types and a standardized nomenclature. An internationally agreed classification of tumours, acceptable alike to physicians, surgeons, radiologists and statisticians, would enable cancer workers in all parts of the world to compare their findings and would facilitate collaboration among them.

In a report published in 1952,[1] a subcommittee on the World Health Organization (WHO) Expert Committee on Health Statistics discussed the general principles that should govern the statistical classification of tumours and agreed that, to ensure the necessary flexibility and ease of coding, three separate classifications were needed according to (1) anatomical site, (2) histological type, and (3) degree of malignancy. A classification according to anatomical site is available in the International Classification of Diseases.[2]

In 1956, the WHO Executive Board passed a resolution[3] requesting the Director-General to explore the possibility that WHO might organize centres in various parts of the world and arrange for the collection of human tissues and their histological classification.

The main purpose of such centres would be to develop histological definitions of cancer types and to facilitate the wide adoption of a uniform nomenclature. The resolution was endorsed by the Tenth World Health Assembly in May 1957.[4]

Since 1958, WHO has established a number of centres concerned with this subject. The result of this endeavour has been the International Histological Classification of Tumours, a multivolumed series whose

---

[1] WHO (1952) WHO Technical Report Series. No. 53, 1952, p. 45
[2] WHO (1977) Manual of the international statistical classification of diseases, injuries, and causes of death. 1975 version. Geneva
[3] WHO (1956) WHO Official Records, No. 68, p. 14 (resolution EB 17.R40)
[4] WHO (1957) WHO Official Records, No. 79, p. 467 (resolution WHA 10.18)

first edition was published between 1967 and 1981. The present revised second edition aims to update the classification, reflecting progress in diagnosis and the relevance of tumour types to clinical and epidemiological features.

Preface to Histological Typing of Female Genital Tract Tumours, Second Edition

The first edition of *Histological Typing of Female Genital Tract Tumours*[1] was the result of a collaborative effort organized by WHO and carried out by the Collaborating Center for the Histological Classification of Female Genital Tract Tumours at the Institute of Pathological Anatomy, Kommunehospitalet, Copenhagen, Denmark. The classification was published in 1975.

The task of updating the classification was given to the Classification and Nomenclature Committee of the International Society of Gynecological Pathologists and its four subcommittees listed on pages V–VIII. Classification proposals were discussed during meetings of the subcommittees and presented orally to the members of the Society during their general meetings. The classifications were finally circulated to the Society members for their suggestions, which were considered and discussed at the final meetings of the subcommittees.

The final classification reflects the present state of knowledge, and modifications are almost certain to be needed as experience accumulates. It is therefore expected that some pathologists may dissent from certain aspects of the classification or terminology adopted in this volume. It is nevertheless hoped that, in the interests of international cooperation and comparability of data, all pathologists will use the classification as put forward. Criticisms and suggestions for its improvement will be welcomed; these should be sent to the World Health Organization, Geneva, Switzerland.

Since many of the tumours and tumour-like conditions in the classification occur in several sites in the female genital tract cross-referencing from one site to another has been done in illustrating these lesions.

The editors and authors are grateful to the International Society of Gynecological Pathologists for its generous financial support for the publication of many of the color photographs.

---

[1] Poulsen HE, Taylor CW, Sobin LH (1975) Histological Typing of Female Genital Tract Tumours. Geneva, World Health Organization (International Histological Classification of Tumours, No. 13)

Contents

Histological Classification of Tumours of the Female Genital Tract

Uterine Corpus

1   **Epithelial Tumours and Related Lesions**

1.1	*Endometrial hyperplasia*	
1.1.1	Simple	72000[a]
1.1.2	Complex (adenomatous)	
1.2	*Atypical endometrial hyperplasia*	72005
1.2.1	Simple	
1.2.2	Complex (adenomatous with atypia)	
1.3	*Endometrial polyp*	76800
1.4	*Endometrial carcinoma*	
1.4.1	Endometrioid	
1.4.1.1	Adenocarcinoma	8380/3
1.4.1.1.1	Secretory (variant)	
1.4.1.1.2	Ciliated cell (variant)	
1.4.1.2	Adenocarcinoma with squamous differentiation ...	8570/3
	(adenoacanthoma; adenosquamous carcinoma)	
1.4.2	Serous adenocarcinoma	8441/3
1.4.3	Clear cell adenocarcinoma	8310/3
1.4.4	Mucinous adenocarcinoma	8480/3
1.4.5	Squamous cell carcinoma	8070/3
1.4.6	Mixed carcinoma	8323/3
1.4.7	Undifferentiated carcinoma	8020/3

2   **Mesenchymal Tumours and Related Lesions**

2.1	*Endometrial stromal tumours*	
2.1.1	Endometrial stromal nodule	8930/0

---

[a] Morphology code of the International Classification of Diseases for Oncology (ICD-O) 1990 and the Systematized Nomenclature of Medicine (SNOMED) 1982

3   Mixed Epithelial and Mesenchymal Tumours

Gestational Trophoblastic Disease

1	**Hydatidiform Mole**	9100/0
1.1	Complete	9100/0
1.2	Partial	9103/0
2	**Invasive Hydatidiform Mole** (chorioadenoma destruens)	9100/1
3	**Choriocarcinoma**	9100/3
4	**Placental Site Trophoblastic Tumour**	9104/1
5	**Miscellaneous Trophoblastic Lesions**	
5.1	Exaggerated placental site	79420
5.2	Placental site nodule and plaque	
6	**Unclassified Trophoblastic Lesions**	

Uterine Cervix

1	**Epithelial Tumours and Related Lesions**	
1.1	*Squamous lesions*	
1.1.1	Squamous papilloma	8052/0
1.1.2	Condyloma acuminatum	76720
1.1.3	Squamous metaplasia	73220
1.1.4	Transitional metaplasia	73260
1.1.5	Squamous atypia	69700
1.1.6	Squamous intraepithelial lesions (dysplasia-carcinoma in situ; cervical intraepithelial neoplasia (CIN))	
1.1.6.1	Mild dysplasia (CIN1)	74006
1.1.6.2	Moderate dysplasia (CIN2)	74007
1.1.6.3	Severe dysplasia (CIN3)	74008
1.1.6.4	Carcinoma in situ (CIN3)	8070/2
1.1.7	Squamous cell carcinoma	8070/3
1.1.7.1	Keratinizing	8071/3
1.1.7.2	Nonkeratinizing	8072/3
1.1.7.3	Verrucous	8051/3
1.1.7.4	Warty (condylomatous)	
1.1.7.5	Papillary	8052/3
1.1.7.6	Lymphoepithelioma-like carcinoma	8082/3

1.2   *Glandular lesions*

1.2.1   Endocervical polyp   76800

1.2.2   Mullerian papilloma

1.2.3   Glandular atypia

1.2.4   Glandular dysplasia   74000

1.2.5   Adenocarcinoma in situ 8140/2

1.2.6   Adenocarcinoma 8140/3

1.2.6.1 Mucinous adenocarcinoma 8480/3

1.2.6.1.1 Endocervical type

1.2.6.1.2 Intestinal type 8144/3

1.2.6.2 Endometrioid adenocarcinoma 8380/3

1.2.6.3 Clear cell adenocarcinoma 8310/3

1.2.6.4 Serous adenocarcinoma 8441/3

1.2.6.5 Mesonephric adenocarcinoma 9110/3

1.3   *Other epithelial tumours*

1.3.1   Adenosquamous carcinoma 8560/3

1.3.2   Glassy cell carcinoma

1.3.3   Adenoid cystic carcinoma 8200/3

1.3.4   Adenoid basal carcinoma 8092/3

1.3.5   Carcinoid tumour 8240/3

1.3.6   Small cell carcinoma 8041/3

1.3.7   Undifferentiated carcinoma 8020/3

2   **Mesenchymal Tumours**

2.1   Leiomyoma 8890/0

2.2   Leiomyosarcoma 8890/3

2.3   Endocervical stromal sarcoma 8930/3

2.4   Sarcoma botryoides

         (embryonal rhabdomyosarcoma) 8910/3

2.5   Endometrioid stromal sarcoma 8930/3

2.6   Alveolar soft-part sarcoma 9581/3

2.7   Others

3   **Mixed Epithelial and Mesenchymal Tumours**

3.1   Adenofibroma 9013/0

3.2   Adenomyoma

3.2.1   Atypical polypoid adenomyoma (variant)

3.3   Adenosarcoma 8933/3

Vagina

1	**Epithelial Tumours and Related Lesions**	
1.1	*Squamous lesions*	
1.1.1	Squamous papilloma	8052/0
1.1.2	Condyloma acuminatum	76720
1.1.3	Transitional metaplasia	73260
1.1.4	Squamous atypia	69700
1.1.5	Squamous intraepithelial lesions (dysplasia – carcinoma in situ; vaginal intraepithelial neoplasia (VAIN))	
1.1.5.1	Mild dysplasia (VAIN1)	74006
1.1.5.2	Moderate dysplasia (VAIN2)	74007
1.1.5.3	Severe dysplasia (VAIN3)	74008
1.1.5.4	Carcinoma in situ (VAIN3)	8070/2
1.1.6	Squamous cell carcinoma	8070/3
1.1.6.1	Keratinizing	8071/3
1.1.6.2	Nonkeratinizing	8072/3
1.1.6.3	Verrucous	8051/3
1.1.6.4	Warty (condylomatous)	
1.2	*Glandular lesions*	
1.2.1	Mullerian papilloma	
1.2.2	Adenosis	74200
1.2.3	Atypical adenosis	
1.2.4	Adenocarcinoma	8140/3
1.2.4.1	Clear cell adenocarcinoma	8310/3
1.2.4.2	Endometrioid adenocarcinoma	8380/3
1.2.4.3	Mucinous adenocarcinoma	8480/3
1.2.4.3.1	Endocervical type	
1.2.4.3.2	Intestinal type	8144/3
1.2.4.4	Mesonephric adenocarcinoma	9110/3
1.3	*Other epithelial tumours*	
1.3.1	Adenosquamous carcinoma	8560/3
1.3.2	Adenoid cystic carcinoma	8200/3
1.3.3	Adenoid basal carcinoma	8092/3
1.3.4	Carcinoid tumour	8240/3
1.3.5	Small cell carcinoma	8041/3
1.3.6	Undifferentiated carcinoma	8020/3

Vulva

Definitions and Explanatory Notes

Uterine Corpus

1 Epithelial Tumours and Related Lesions

1.1 Endometrial Hyperplasia

A proliferation of endometrial glands without cytologic atypia.

1.1.1 Simple (Figs. 1, 2)

1.1.2 Complex (Adenomatous) (Figs. 3, 4)

1.2 Atypical Endometrial Hyperplasia (Figs. 5, 6)

A proliferation of endometrial glands with cytologic atypia.

1.2.1 Simple

1.2.2 Complex (Adenomatous with Atypia)

Endometrial hyperplasia may be focal or diffuse; cytologic atypia in hyperplastic glands is typically focal. Hyperplastic endometrial glands are usually of proliferative type, but a focal or diffuse secretory change, metaplastic or related changes, or both may be present as well.

Although the endometrial glands are usually increased in number per unit volume in simple hyperplasia, the endometrial stroma is typically hyperplastic as well. The glands may be cystically dilated and slightly to moderately crowded. In complex hyperplasia the glands are markedly crowded and typically have irregular outlines, resulting in a complex pattern. Cytologic atypia is characterized by significant nuclear abnormalities, including loss of polarity, and may be superimposed on either simple or complex hyperplasia in atypical hyperplasia.

The above terminology was selected because of the confusion in the literature regarding the widely used designation "adenomatous". Some authors have employed this term to denote architecturally abnormal but cytologically typical endometrial glands and others have used it to signify architecturally abnormal and cytologically atypical glands. The term "atypical adenomatous hyperplasia" has also appeared in the literature. In the alternative terminology, given in parentheses, the word "adenomatous" designates an architectural (complex-glandular) abnormality only; cytologic atypia, if present, must be noted additionally.

Endometrial hyperplasia must be distinguished from an endometrial polyp, glandular alterations accompanying endometritis, epithelial metaplasias, normal or slightly altered cycling endometrium, glandular alterations caused by pregnancy and progestin therapy, and adenocarcinoma.

Atypical endometrial hyperplasia is capable of progression to carcinoma if not adequately treated. The malignant potential of endometrial hyperplasia without cytologic atypia is considerably less.

1.3 Endometrial Polyp (Figs. 7, 8)

A benign nodular protrusion above the endometrial surface consisting of endometrial glands and stroma that is typically at least focally fibrous and contains thick-walled blood vessels.

Endometrial polyps are common, may be single or multiple, and vary in size from incidental microscopic findings to bulky masses that may prolapse through the external os; polyps are often pedunculated. The glands in endometrial polyps are usually inactive or weakly proliferative, but they may show secretory change, various forms of metaplasia, or hyperplasia. Carcinomas and other malignant tumours may arise within endometrial polyps.

1.4 Endometrial Carcinoma

1.4.1 Endometrioid

1.4.1.1 Adenocarcinoma (Figs. 9–12)

A carcinoma containing glands resembling those of the normal endometrium.

1.4.1.1.1 Secretory (Variant) (Fig. 13)

An endometrioid adenocarcinoma containing glands resembling those of an early secretory endometrium.

1.4.1.1.2 Ciliated Cell (Variant) (Fig. 14)

An endometrioid adenocarcinoma in which the majority of the cells bear cilia.

Endometrioid adenocarcinoma is the most common form of endometrial carcinoma. The glands show varying degrees of cytologic atypia, are often uniform in size and shape, and invade the stroma. When the tumour has a papillary, villoglandular pattern (Fig. 12) it must be distinguished from serous papillary and clear cell papillary adenocarcinomas, which are generally more highly aggressive.

The glandular component of all endometrioid carcinomas is graded as follows:

Grade 1: 5 % or less nonsquamous solid growth pattern
Grade 2: 6 %–50 % nonsquamous solid growth pattern
Grade 3: More than 50 % of a nonsquamous solid growth pattern
Notable nuclear atypia inappropriately severe for the architectural grade of the tumour raises the grade of otherwise grade 1 or grade 2 tumours by one.

1.4.1.2 Adenocarcinoma with Squamous Differentiation (Adenoacanthoma; Adenosquamous Carcinoma) (Figs. 15–17)

An endometrioid adenocarcinoma in which there is focal differentiation into benign or malignant appearing squamous epithelium

Adenocarcinomas with squamous differentiation are graded according to the grade of the glandular component. Because endometrioid carcinomas may contain significant areas of solid growth of either glandular or squamous epithelial cells, strict criteria must be applied for identification of the squamous element in adenocarcinomas with squamous differentiation. A solid focus of tumour in an endometrioid carcinoma should be considered glandular unless at least one of the following features of squamous differentiation is present: (1) keratinization demonstrated by standard staining techniques; (2) intercellular bridges; (3) three or more of the following four features: sheet-like growth without gland formation or nuclear palisading; sharp cell margins; eosinophilic, dense or glassy cytoplasm; a decreased nuclear-cytoplasmic ratio in comparison with other foci in the tumour.

Once squamous differentiation is identified by the above criteria, the squamous cells may be classified as histologically malignant (adenosquamous carcinoma) as opposed to histologically benign (adenoacanthoma) if they have one or more of the following features: standard cytologic features of malignancy; mitotic figures; destructive stromal infiltration.

Malignant squamous elements in these tumours do not require grading. The designation "adenocarcinoma with squamous differentiation", with grading of the glandular component only, is currently preferred over the subdivision of these tumours into "adenoacanthoma" and "adenosquamous carcinoma".

1.4.2 Serous Adenocarcinoma (Fig. 18)

An adenocarcinoma characterized by a complex pattern of papillae with cellular budding and the frequent presence of psammoma bodies.

Serous adenocarcinoma is recognized by criteria similar to those used to diagnose serous adenocarcinoma of the ovary. The papillae have broad fibrovascular connective tissue cores lined by irregularly stratified and generally poorly differentiated cells that form secondary papillae and cellular buds. The nuclei are generally highly atypical, foci of necrosis are frequently seen, psammoma bodies are detectable in approximately one third of the cases, and solid sheets of undifferentiated cells are commonly present. The tumour characteristically infiltrates the myometrium within lymphatic or blood vascular channels and is often widely disseminated at the time of diagnosis.

1.4.3 Clear Cell Adenocarcinoma (see Vagina, Figs. 148–150)

An adenocarcinoma composed mainly of clear cells or hobnail cells arranged in solid, tubulocystic, or papillary patterns or a combination of these patterns.

The clear cell adenocarcinoma also has a tendency to early dissemination.

1.4.4 Mucinous Adenocarcinoma (Fig. 19)

An adenocarcinoma in which most of the tumour cells contain abundant intracytoplasmic mucin.

Mucinous adenocarcinomas are usually well differentiated and may resemble mucinous adenocarcinomas of the cervix. Accordingly, it is important to rule out the possibility of an endocervical adenocarcinoma extending to the endometrium before one makes the diagnosis of a primary mucinous adenocarcinoma of the endometrium. It is also important to distinguish the latter from mucinous metaplasia of the endometrium, which is usually accomplished by the finding of stromal invasion, cellular stratification, and nuclear atypia in mucinous adenocarcinoma.

1.4.5 Squamous Cell Carcinoma

A carcinoma composed of squamous cells of varying degrees of differentiation.

Squamous cell carcinoma of the endometrium is rare. Before making the diagnosis, one must exclude a squamous cell carcinoma of the cervix extending to the endometrium and adenocarcinoma of the endometrium with squamous differentiation in which the squamous component is predominant.

1.4.6 Mixed Carcinoma

A carcinoma (other than adenocarcinoma with squamous differentiation) in which one or more additional types account for at least 10 % of the entire tumour.

The diagnosis of a mixed carcinoma is optimally made on examination of a hysterectomy specimen, but if only a smaller specimen is available, any amount of a second tumour category suffices for the diagnosis. When a carcinoma is classified as mixed, the major and minor types and their relative proportions should be specified.

1.4.7 Undifferentiated Carcinoma

A carcinoma with minimal or no differentiation into any of the above cell types.

Undifferentiated carcinoma includes large cell, giant cell, spindle cell, and small cell forms. The small cell undifferentiated carcinoma may contain argyrophil cells and should be distinguished from endometrial carcinomas of other types, which may also contain small or large numbers of argyrophil cells. The latter tumours should be designated as one or another of the tumour types already described. Their content of argyrophil cells may be commented on separately, but the term "argyrophil cell carcinoma" is not warranted.

Other types of carcinoma that occur more commonly in other sites have been reported rarely in the endometrium. It is recommended that "glassy cell carcinoma" be classified as a subtype of adenocarcinoma with squamous differentiation, "verrucous carcinoma" as a subtype of squamous cell carcinoma, and "mucoepidermoid carcinoma" as a variant of mucinous adenocarcinoma.

2 Mesenchymal Tumours and Related Lesions

2.1 Endometrial Stromal Tumours

2.1.1 Endometrial Stromal Nodule (Figs. 20, 21)

A benign tumour of cells resembling endometrial stromal cells, having a pushing interface with adjacent endometrium or myometrium and lacking vascular space invasion.

2.1.2 Endometrial Stromal Sarcoma, Low Grade (Endolymphatic Stromal Myosis) (Figs. 22, 23)

A sarcoma composed of cells resembling normal endometrial stromal cells, invading the myometrium, usually invading its vascular spaces, and occasionally extending into extrauterine vessels.

2.1.3 Endometrial Stromal Sarcoma, High Grade (Fig. 24)

A poorly differentiated sarcoma without specific features or heterologous elements but with an infiltrating pattern that suggests an origin from endometrial stromal cells.

Only the stromal nodule and low grade sarcoma are composed of cells with a close resemblance to normal endometrial stromal cells. These two tumour types may appear identical at high magnification, with the only difference between them being the pushing border of the stromal nodule and the infiltration into adjacent tissues and vessels by low grade stromal sarcoma. Foci of hyalinization, foam cell change, smooth muscle metaplasia, glands and sex cord-like structures may be seen in both stromal nodules and low grade stromal sarcomas. The sex cord-like cells typically contain nuclei similar to those of the obvious stromal cells, distinguishing tumours containing these structures from carcinomas and from adenosarcomas with benign or atypical glands.

Since the distinction between a benign stromal nodule and a low grade stromal sarcoma is made solely on the basis of the character of its border, a definitive diagnosis can be made only rarely prior to hysterectomy. Thus, a diagnosis such as "stromal tumour, final diagnosis pending" is appropriate for a curettage specimen.

High grade stromal sarcomas share with the low grade type an infiltrative margin, but otherwise differ in appearance. They may be composed of pleomorphic cells with numerous mitotic figures that may bear little resemblance to benign endometrial stromal cells.

2.2 Smooth Muscle Tumours

2.2.1 Leiomyoma (Figs. 25, 26)

A benign neoplasm composed of smooth muscle cells with a variable amount of fibrous stroma.

The leiomyoma is the most common tumour of the uterus and one of the most common neoplasms in women. It is seen predominantly during the reproductive years and may be single or multiple, and microscopic or very large; it may be an incidental finding or cause symptoms. Numerous variations in the appearance of leiomyomas are seen in addition to those specifically designated in the classification. Particularly common are degenerative changes, which include hemorrhage, necrosis, hyalinization, edema, and myxoid change. These changes may occur in malignant as well as benign smooth muscle tumours and their presence should not alter the diagnosis.

2.2.1.1 Cellular (Variant) (Fig. 27)

A leiomyoma that is significantly more cellular than the adjacent myometrium.

Since most leiomyomas are more cellular than the adjacent myometrium, "significantly" has been included in the definition. Tumours so designated should account for no more than 5 % of all uterine leiomyomas. In the absence of atypia and prominent mitotic activity, the cellular variant does not have a malignant potential.

2.2.1.2 Epithelioid (Variant) (Figs. 28, 29)

A leiomyoma composed of cells resembling epithelial cells.

Three terms have been used in the literature to designate microscopic subtypes of epithelioid leiomyoma. "Leiomyoblastoma" has been restricted by some authors to epithelioid leiomyomas composed of cells containing abundant eosinophilic cytoplasm. "Clear cell leiomyoma" has been employed for tumours containing a preponderance of cells with abundant clear cytoplasm. "Plexiform leiomyoma" refers to tumours in which the neoplastic cells have an epithelial-like plexiform architecture; microscopic myometrial and occasionally endometrial tumours of this type have been designated "plexiform tumourlets".

The myometrial location of most of these tumours, the presence of foci of more typical smooth muscle differentiation, and the use of connective tissue stains, immunohistochemical techniques, and electron microscopy may aid in their diagnosis.

2.2.1.3 Bizarre (Variant) (Fig. 30)

A leiomyoma containing giant cells with pleomorphic nuclei and little or no mitotic activity.

The bizarre leiomyoma is also known as "symplastic" or "pleomorphic" leiomyoma. Unlike most leiomyosarcomas, this tumour is often extensively hyalinized.

2.2.1.4 Lipoleiomyoma (Variant) (Fig. 31)

A leiomyoma that contains mature adipocytes and smooth muscle cells.

Unlike other leiomyomas the lipoleiomyoma is seen most commonly in postmenopausal women.

2.2.2 Smooth Muscle Tumour of Uncertain Malignant Potential

A smooth muscle tumour that cannot be diagnosed reliably as benign or malignant on the basis of generally applied criteria.

This tumour can best be defined against the background of the definitions of leiomyoma, leiomyosarcoma, and their variants. When the diagnosis of uncertain malignant potential is made, the reason for the diagnosis should be specified (e. g., marked cellularity and atypia but few mitotic figures).

2.2.3 Leiomyosarcoma (Figs. 32, 33)

A malignant tumour of smooth muscle cells.

Leiomyosarcomas are rare, occurring most frequently in post-menopausal women. The typical leiomyosarcoma is easily distinguished from a leiomyoma by its dense cellularity, prominent nuclear pleomorphism, frequent mitotic figures including atypical forms, and infiltrative borders. Any morphologic variant of leiomyoma may also be encountered in leiomyosarcoma.

2.2.3.1 Epithelioid (Variant)

A leiomyosarcoma composed of cells resembling epithelial cells.

2.2.3.2 Myxoid (Variant)

An infiltrating smooth muscle tumour in which myxoid material separates the tumour cells.

This tumour may have little or no nuclear atypia or mitotic activity and is diagnosed mainly on the basis of its infiltrative margins.

2.2.4 Other smooth muscle tumours

This category includes tumours that reflect variations in the growth patterns of leiomyomas.

2.2.4.1 Metastasizing Leiomyoma

A benign appearing smooth muscle tumour of the uterus that is found to have metastasized to extrauterine sites such as the lung or pelvic lymph nodes, usually many years after hysterectomy.

This diagnosis can be made only if metastasis has occurred and both the uterine and the extrauterine tumour show no microscopic evidence of malignancy. Whether the extrauterine tumours are metastatic or reflect multifocal tumour formation has been debated in some cases.

2.2.4.2 Intravenous Leiomyomatosis (Fig. 34)

A cytologically benign uterine smooth muscle tumour that has invaded veins.

This type of leiomyoma extends continuously into uterine veins, often extrauterine veins, and occasionally the right chambers of the heart, and may be fatal. The lesion may arise from smooth muscle in vein walls or from myometrial smooth muscle. Histologically atypical variants occur, but if the tumour shows significant nuclear atypicality and mitotic activity, it is preferably classified as a leiomyosarcoma.

2.2.4.3 Diffuse Leiomyomatosis (Fig. 35)

A rare condition in which myriads of small leiomyomas coalese to replace most of the myometrium.

2.3 Mixed Endometrial Stromal and Smooth Muscle Tumours (Fig. 36)

Tumours showing both endometrial stromal and smooth muscle differentiation recognizable on light microscopic examination.

Tumours of this type may be benign, malignant, or of uncertain malignant potential. Determination of their malignant potential should be based on evaluation of their more malignant component. Immunohistochemical evidence of smooth muscle differentiation in an endometrial stromal tumour is not sufficient evidence by itself for the diagnosis of a mixed tumour, but smooth muscle differentiation must be also apparent on routine histological staining.

2.4 Adenomatoid Tumour (Figs. 37, 38)

A benign tumour of the uterine serosa and myometrium originating from mesothelium and forming gland-like structures.

This tumour appears as either a localized or a diffuse lesion of the myometrium; the gland-like structures are lined by flat to cuboidal cells with bland nuclei. Despite its frequent lack of circumscription, this tumour is benign.

2.5 Other Mesenchymal Tumours

This category comprises generally unrelated tumours, all of which are more common in extrauterine locations. Examples are haemangioma, lymphangioma, lipoma, rhabdomyosarcoma, chondrosarcoma, osteosarcoma, and liposarcoma.

2.5.1 Homologous

A tumour composed entirely of mesenchymal tissue types that are normally present in the uterus.

2.5.2 Heterologous

A tumour containing one or more mesenchymal tissue types not normally encountered in the uterus, such as cartilage and striated muscle.

3 Mixed Epithelial and Mesenchymal Tumours

3.1 Benign

3.1.1 Adenofibroma (see Cervix, Fig. 128)

A benign tumour of the endometrium composed of epithelium of mullerian type and a fibroblastic or endometrial type stroma.

The adenofibroma is rare and typically shows club-shaped papillae and glands lined by glandular epithelium of mullerian type and a bland stroma that is usually fibroblastic; squamous metaplasia of the glandular epithelium may occur.

3.1.2 Adenomyoma

A benign tumour composed of endometrial type glands and smooth muscle.

3.1.2.1 Atypical Polypoid Adenomyoma (Variant) (Figs. 39, 40)

A polypoid adenomyoma composed of intimately admixed atypical endometrial glands and smooth muscle.

In the atypical polypoid adenomyoma, architecturally and cytologically atypical endometrial glands, usually showing focal squamous morular differentiation, are distributed in a stroma consisting of fascicles of bland smooth muscle. The tumour occurs predominantly in the lower uterine segment of relatively young women and should not be confused with an adenosarcoma, carcinosarcoma, or well differentiated endometrioid carcinoma invading the myometrium.

3.2 Malignant

3.2.1 Adenosarcoma (Figs. 41, 42)

A mixed tumour composed of benign or atypical epithelium of mullerian type and a malignant appearing stroma.

This tumour usually has the same pattern of growth as an adenofibroma, and well differentiated forms may be difficult to distinguish from the latter. The stromal component, however, is typically more cellular, especially in a layer immediately adjacent to the epithelial component, and shows varying degrees of atypia and mitotic activity. In some cases, the stromal component contains heterologous elements such as cartilage or striated muscle. Adenosarcomas are similar both in their histological features and their behaviour to cystosarcoma phyllodes of the breast, and typically are of low grade malignancy. Adenosarcomas in which un-interrupted fields of pure sarcoma account for 20 % or more of the total tumour area (adenosarcomas with sarcomatous overgrowth) have a higher potential for recurrence and metastasis than tumours without these features. Although locally recurrent tumours may contain both glandular and stromal components, metastases have consisted of the stromal component only.

3.2.1.1 Homologous (Fig. 41)

3.2.1.2 Heterologous (Fig. 42)

3.2.2 Carcinofibroma

A very rare tumour with a malignant epithelial component and a benign fi-bromatous component.

3.2.3 Carcinosarcoma (Malignant Mesodermal Mixed Tumour; Malignant Mullerian Mixed Tumour)

A malignant tumour composed of both carcinoma and sarcoma.

The carcinosarcoma is the most common mixed tumour. The diagnosis requires the presence of indisputably malignant epithelial and stromal elements. Carcinoma with spindle cell differentiation should be excluded on routine histological examination; immunohistochemical and ultrastructural evidence suggesting that the tumour is metaplastic carcinoma, in the absence of convincing evidence for the latter on routine staining, does not exclude the diagnosis of carcinosarcoma.

Although some authors have used the term "malignant mullerian mixed tumour" for those neoplasms containing heterologous elements, such as cartilage, skeletal muscle, and bone, and "carcinosarcoma" for those tumours lacking such components, these two designations are generally used synonymously at the present time, with the word "homologous" or "heterologous" appended to them. There appears to be very little, if any, difference in behaviour between the two subtypes of carcinosarcoma.

3.2.3.1 Homologous (Fig. 43)

3.2.3.2 Heterologous (Figs. 44, 45)

4 Miscellaneous Tumours

4.1 Sex Cord-like Tumours (Figs. 46, 47)

Uterine tumours composed predominantly or entirely of epithelial-like structures resembling those seen in sex cord-stromal tumours of the ovary.

Foci of sex cord-like differentiation may be seen as minor components of both endometrial stromal and smooth muscle tumours of the uterus. Rare uterine tumours that are composed predominantly of sex cord-like structures should be classified separately. Evaluation of the pushing or infiltrating nature of the tumour border, nuclear abnormalities and vascular space invasion are important in predicting the behaviour of the tumour.

4.2 Tumours of Germ Cell Type

Primary tumours having morphologic features of germ cell tumours of the ovary.

Rarely, teratomas and other malignant tumours of germ cell type such as yolk sac tumour are primary in the uterine corpus.

4.3 Neuroectodermal Tumours (Fig. 48)

Neoplasms showing neuroectodermal differentiation.

These tumours are extremely rare. Those of glial type (uterine gliomas) can be distinguished from benign glial tissue in the endometrium by their invasion of the myometrium.

4.4 Lymphoma and Leukemia (see Vagina, Fig. 157)

Although most malignant lymphomas of the uterine corpus are a manifestation of disseminated disease, on rare occasions the uterus may be the first known site of a lymphoma. The classification of lymphomas of the uterus is similar to that in more common locations. Myometrial invasion is an important feature distinguishing malignant lymphomas from lymphoma-like lesions (see p. 30).

4.5 Others

Many other types of tumour may manifest themselves initially or exclusively in the uterine corpus. The classification of such tumours should follow the principles established for their classification in more common sites of occurrence.

5 Secondary Tumours (Fig. 49)

Tumours that have extended directly or metastasized to the uterine corpus.
These tumours are encountered uncommonly in surgical specimens, in which they may be confused with primary uterine neoplasms, and are seen more often at autopsy. The possibility of a secondary tumour should always be considered when one encounters a uterine tumour that does not fit clearly into one of the primary tumour categories in this classification. The diagnosis of a secondary tumour may be difficult to make if the presence of a primary extrauterine tumour is not known to the pathologist.

6 Tumour-like Lesions

6.1 Epithelial Metaplastic and Related Changes

Nonneoplastic lesions of one or more types in which endometrial epithelium is replaced, usually focally, by another type of epithelium.
The main significance of these lesions is their tendency to be confused with an endometrial hyperplastic or neoplastic lesion. Confounding their interpretation is their occasional occurrence in association with hyperplastic or neoplastic instead of otherwise normal endometrial epithelium.

6.1.1 Squamous Metaplasia, Including Morule Formation
(Fig. 50)

In squamous metaplasia, the metaplastic epithelium may resemble native or metaplastic squamous epithelium of the uterine cervix and, in the morular form, hyperplasia of reserve cells of the cervix. The diagnosis of adenocarcinoma with squamous differentiation should not be made unless the glandular component of the lesion is clearly malignant.

6.1.2 Mucinous Metaplasia, Including Intestinal Type (Fig. 51)

Mucinous metaplasia is characterized by conversion of endometrial epithelium to an epithelium composed largely or completely of mucin-containing cells; the mucinous epithelium resembles endocervical or much less commonly intestinal epithelium. This change is usually limited to a small number of glands and must be distinguished from mucinous adenocarcinomas of endometrial, endocervical, or extrauterine origin.

6.1.3 Ciliated Cell Metaplasia (see Cervix, Fig. 141)

Ciliated cell metaplasia is frequently referred to as "tubal metaplasia", but the metaplastic epithelium usually does not include all the cell types seen in normal adult fallopian tube epithelium. Since a few ciliated cells are common in normal endometrium, the diagnosis of metaplasia should be made only when one or more endometrial glands are lined predominantly by ciliated cells.

6.1.4 Hobnail Cell Metaplasia (Fig. 52)

Hobnail cell metaplasia, in which the nuclei have a bulbous shape and are situated in the apical portion of the cell, is frequent in regenerating endometrial epithelium and rare in other situations. The cells are differentiated from those encountered in clear cell adenocarcinoma by their bland nuclei and their occurrence in surface epithelium or glands that lack the architectural features of adenocarcinoma. Hobnail cells are also encountered in the Arias-Stella change (see p. 28).

6.1.5 Clear Cell Change (Fig. 53)

In clear cell change one or more endometrial glands are lined by cells with voluminous clear cytoplasm containing glycogen. Although the lesion may resemble clear cell or secretory adenocarcinoma the architectural features of carcinoma are absent, and the nuclei are uniform and cytologically bland. The lesion is seen most frequently in association with pregnancy.

6.1.6 Eosinophilic Cell Metaplasia, Including Oncocytic (Fig. 54)

In eosinophilic cell change the glands are lined by cells with eosinophilic, sometimes granular (oncocytic) cytoplasm. In contrast to some forms of atypical hyperplasia with eosinophilic cell change, the cells are not stratified and the nuclei are not atypical.

6.1.7 Surface Syncytial Change (Fig. 55)

6.1.8 Papillary Change (Fig. 56)

Surface syncytial change and papillary change are both common, may be extensive, and frequently coexist. Indistinct cytoplasmic margins, microcystic degenerative change, and infiltration by neutrophils are characteristic of surface syncytial change. In both lesions, the nuclei are bland, aiding in their distinction from serous and other types of adenocarcinoma.

6.1.9 Arias-Stella Change (Figs. 57, 58)

A transformation of endometrial glandular epithelial cells into hobnail cells with nuclear enlargement and hyperchromatism occurring mainly during pregnancy.

Arias-Stella change is associated with pregnancy and other conditions of increased progestational stimulation. In the typical form, the glandular epithelium is typically composed of hobnail cells and may be accompanied by hypersecretion. The absence of architectural features of carcinoma, the presence of other gestational changes, the rarity of mitotic figures, and the clinical history all help to distinguish this change from clear cell adenocarcinoma.

6.2 Stromal Metaplastic and Related Changes

Changes in which endometrial stroma is focally replaced by nonneoplastic mesenchymal or other tissues that are not encountered in normal endometrium.

These conditions are rarer than epithelial metaplastic and related changes, do not have the propensity of the latter to be admixed, and are less likely to be confused with malignant tumours. In the case of osseous metaplasia, cartilaginous metaplasia, and fatty change, the major pitfall is the misdiagnosis of adenosarcoma or carcinosarcoma with a heterologous component and, in the case of smooth muscle metaplasia, the misdiagnosis of endometrial stromal sarcoma or leiomyosarcoma. The focal nature of these changes, their bland cytologic appearance, and their lack of association with histologically malignant epithelial or homologous stromal elements should suffice to exclude a malignant diagnosis.

6.2.1 Smooth Muscle Metaplasia

6.2.2 Osseous Metaplasia and Retention of Fetal Bone

6.2.3 Cartilaginous Metaplasia and Retention of Fetal Cartilage

6.2.4 Adipocyte Metaplasia

6.2.5 Retention of Fetal Glial Tissue

Glial tissue typically occurs alone, is mature, and, unlike a glioma, does not invade the myometrium. Glial tissue, like osseous and cartilaginous tissue, may be the residuum of a clinically silent abortion.

6.2.6 Foam Cell Change (Fig. 59)

Foam cell change, an accumulation of lipid vacuoles within the cytoplasm of endometrial stromal cells, is seen most frequently in the stroma of an endometrial carcinoma but may also be encountered in the stroma in endometrial hyperplasia, endometrial polyps, and otherwise unremarkable endometria. Foam cell change can also be seen in stromal nodules, stromal sarcomas, and adenosarcomas. Another type of foam cell that is occasionally present in the endometrium, particularly in association with chronic inflammation, is the foamy histiocyte.

6.3 Adenomyosis (Fig. 60)

A nonneoplastic condition in which islands of benign endometrial glands and stroma are present in the myometrium, mainly in its inner portion.

Since the junction between endometrium and myometrium is often irregular in the normal uterus, the presence of intramyometrial islands of endometrium discontinuous from the overlying endometrium is necessary for the diagnosis of adenomyosis. Some experts require that such islands should be at least one low power field from the endometrial-myometrial junction to warrant the diagnosis. Serial sections have usually demonstrated continuity of adenomyotic islands with the endometrium. The glands of adenomyosis are usually of basalis type or in the proliferative phase, but may show secretory changes. When adenomyosis is extensive, the uterus may be moderately to markedly enlarged. Although adenomyosis is neither a neoplastic nor a precancerous condition, endometrial hyperplasia and carcinoma may penetrate into or arise within it. It is important to distinguish carcinoma involving adenomyotic islands from true invasion of the myometrium by carcinoma.

6.4 Epithelial Cysts of Myometrium

Intramyometrial cysts lined by histologically benign epithelium without surrounding endometrial stroma.

6.5 Chronic Endometritis (Fig. 61)

Lymphocytes are a normal component of the endometrium, and their presence does not warrant a diagnosis of chronic endometritis (even when they are numerous and forming follicles) unless plasma cells are also identified within the infiltrate. In the presence of a chronic inflammatory infiltrate in the endometrium, particularly if it is granulomatous, the endometrial glands may show atypical reactive changes that may be misinterpreted as hyperplasia or even adenocarcinoma. A marked plasmacytic response and granulomas are only rarely found within the stroma of an endometrial carcinoma; thus, the combination of these stromal changes and a worrisome endometrial glandular proliferation is more likely to represent the reactive atypia of chronic endometritis than atypical hyperplasia or carcinoma.

6.6 Lymphoma-like Lesions (Fig. 62)

Nonneoplastic proliferations of lymphoid tissue that resemble malignant lymphoma.

Rarely the stroma is massively infiltrated by lymphoid cells, some of which may be immature, including immunoblasts. Other inflammatory cells such as plasma cells and polymorphonuclear leukocytes are typically present within the infiltrate, a gross mass is seldom present, and myometrial invasion is absent in contrast to the findings in a malignant lymphoma. Massive benign lymphoid infiltrates are also encountered rarely within uterine leiomyomas.

6.7 Inflammatory Pseudotumour (Fig. 63)

A nonneoplastic mass characterized by spindle cells of myofibroblastic type, plasma cells, and other inflammatory cells.

Inflammatory pseudotumours of the uterus are rare and duplicate similar lesions in other sites in their histological appearance. They present clinically as solitary leiomyoma-like masses and must be distinguished from low grade sarcomas.

6.8 Others

Numerous tumour-like lesions are included in this category. Xanthogranulomatous endometritis and malakoplakia are unusual variants of chronic endometritis. A postoperative spindle cell nodule (see Vagina, Figs. 160, 161) has been reported in the uterine corpus. Epithelial and stromal atypias after radiation therapy also belong in this category.

Gestational Trophoblastic Disease

The taxonomy of trophoblastic lesions has reached an important crossroad in its evolution. On the one hand, the necessity of a morphologic classification has been questioned since the current management of gestational trophoblastic disease is largely medical and is often conducted in the absence of a histological diagnosis. On the other hand, the importance of histological diagnosis is underscored by recent light microscopic studies, complemented by immunocytochemical and cytogenetic techniques, that have drawn attention to two types of trophoblastic lesion of uncertain behaviour. One of these, the partial hydatidiform mole, had not been recognized previously as a distinct entity but now has been shown to have characteristic morphologic and cytogenetic features, justifying its separation from the complete (classic) mole.

   The other recently described trophoblastic lesion, the placental site trophoblastic tumour, had been regarded erroneously as a malignant mesenchymal tumour, a benign trophoblastic lesion, or an atypical choriocarcinoma in the past. Even now it may be difficult in some cases to distinguish a placental site trophoblastic tumour from a nonneoplastic but exuberant proliferation of trophoblast at the implantation site on the basis of existent histological criteria.

   A morphologic classification is required for standardized reporting of data. The classification that follows is intended to furnish a general frame of reference for the histopathology of trophoblastic disease. Definitions and descriptions are provided to supplement the classification and are not intended to be a comprehensive treatise on the subject. Nonetheless, the nature of the disease processes and the limitations of current histological methods make it almost impossible to formulate statements about trophoblastic lesions without adding qualifiers and noting exceptions.

Morphologic and Biologic Characteristics of Trophoblast (Fig. 64)

Normal trophoblast has certain unique biological characteristics that are more akin to those of a malignant tumour than to those of normal tissue. From its location surrounding the blastocyst trophoblast extends centrifugally to invade the endometrium, myometrium and spiral arteries, establishing the uteroplacental circulation. As a result of this vascular invasion, trophoblast disseminates widely in the blood stream, notably to the lungs, throughout normal pregnancy, disappearing after parturition.

The trophoblast that covers the chorionic villi is termed "villous trophoblast". Trophoblast in other sites within the uterus is designated "extravillous trophoblast". Extravillous trophoblast forms the trophoblastic columns traversing the intervillous space from the bases of the anchoring villi; infiltrates the decidua surrounding the blastocyst to form the trophoblastic shell, part of which is sustained as the epithelial layer of the chorion laeve; invades the spiral arteries of the placental bed; and infiltrates the myometrium beneath the implantation site.

Trophoblast is composed of a heterogeneous population of cells among which three morphologically distinct types have been characterized: cytotrophoblast, syncytiotrophoblast, and intermediate trophoblast. Cytotrophoblast is composed of uniform, polygonal to oval epithelial cells with single, round nuclei, scanty, clear to granular cytoplasm and well defined cell borders. Mitotic activity is brisk, consistent with the germinative role of this layer. Syncytiotrophoblast is composed of multinucleated cells with abundant amphophilic or eosinophilic cytoplasm, which, in the first 2 weeks of gestation, contains vacuoles of varying size, some of which form lacunae. A distinct brush border often covers the free surfaces of the cells. Mitotic activity is absent in syncytiotrophoblast as it is the most differentiated form of trophoblast. Intermediate trophoblast consists mostly of mononucleate cells that are larger than cytotrophoblastic cells but multinucleate forms also occur. Intermediate trophoblastic cells are round or polygonal in villous trophoblast and may be spindle-shaped in extravillous trophoblast. They have well defined cell membranes and abundant amphophilic or eosinophilic cytoplasm.

Their nuclei vary from round and lobate to ovoid and have irregularly dispersed chromatin; mitotic figures are rare. Intermediate trophoblastic cells share some characteristics with cytotrophoblastic and syncytiotrophoblastic cells but have light microscopic, ultrastructural, biochemical, and functional features distinct from those of the latter two cell types.

1 Hydatidiform Mole

A trophoblastic lesion characterized by hydropic swelling of chorionic villi and trophoblastic proliferation without evidence of myometrial invasion or vascular deportation.

1.1 Complete (Figs. 65–67)

A hydatidiform mole involving most of the chorionic villi and typically having a diploid karyotype.

The designation "complete hydatidiform mole" applies to most of the lesions previously termed "hydatidiform mole". Although a few small villi are usually present, most of the villi display cistern formation, characterized by a prominent acellular central space. The villi are usually avascular, although occasionally attenuated vascular spaces may be present.

All complete moles display some degree of trophoblastic proliferation on the villous surfaces, which is circumferential but haphazard. The proliferation may be marked, affecting most of the villi, or only minimal and focal, emphasizing the need for thorough sampling. The trophoblastic population is composed of all three types of trophoblastic cells in varying proportions. Cellular atypia of the trophoblast, characterized by enlarged, pleomorphic and hyperchromatic nuclei, varies in degree but is almost uniformly present. Since all patients with complete moles, irrespective of their histological characteristics, should be followed and managed in the same manner, histological grading is unnecessary.

The karyotype of the complete mole is usually 46XX but occasionally it is 46XY. Both sets of chromosomes are paternal in origin, derived from the fertilization of an "empty" ovum either by a single X-bearing sperm that duplicates its haploid chromosomal complement or by two sperm. An embryo or fetus is absent; the presence of a fetus is evidence of a twin gestation.

1.2 Partial (Figs. 68–70)

A hydatidiform mole with two populations of chorionic villi, one of normal size, and the other, hydropic with focal trophoblastic proliferation; the lesion typically has a triploid karyotype.

In contrast to the complete mole the hydropic swelling in the partial mole is focal and typically less marked; also, cistern formation is less pronounced and more focal. The chorionic villi often have a scalloped outline in contrast to their round, distended appearance in the complete mole; trophoblastic pseudoinclusions are also frequently seen within the hydropic villi. Although scalloping and trophoblastic pseudoinclusions are very useful diagnostic features of the partial mole, each of them is occasionally observed in other trophoblastic disorders as well. In addition, the villous stroma of the partial mole frequently undergoes fibrosis in contrast to the complete mole, in which mesenchymal edema is accompanied by cistern formation. The villous capillaries of the partial mole frequently contain nucleated red blood cells, and the trophoblast covering the villi is usually only focally and mildly hyperplastic. The cellular population of the partial mole is composed of cytotrophoblast and syncytiotrophoblast. The latter typically forms focal aggregates on the villous surface; intermediate trophoblast is rarely encountered.

The partial mole usually has a triploid karyotype, typically 69XXY but occasionally 69XXX and very rarely 69XYY. The chromosomes are derived from the fertilization of a normal ovum by two haploid sperm. A fetus or fetal membranes are often present but may require careful examination to detect since early fetal death (at 8–9 weeks menstrual age) is the rule.

The biologic behaviour of the partial mole has not been fully delineated although the risk of development of persistent trophoblastic disease appears to be much less than that for the complete mole. Rare examples of invasive partial mole have occurred but no fully authenticated case of choriocarcinoma associated with a partial mole has been recorded.

At times an hydropic abortus (blighted ovum) may be difficult to distinguish from a partial mole (Figs. 71, 72). In contrast to a complete or partial mole, macroscopic villous swelling is absent in the hydropic abortus, and cistern formation is rare. The important difference between the hydatidiform mole and the hydropic abortus, however, resides in the trophoblast. The swollen villi of the common abortus are typically surrounded by attenuated trophoblast. When trophoblastic proliferation occurs under these circumstances, it is orderly, centrifugal, and polar. These features are not characteristic of a hydatidiform mole. Moreover, trophoblastic atypia is not a feature of an hydropic abortus; when present, it suggests a hydatidiform mole. In the majority of cases of an hydropic abortus the embryo or fetus is absent.

2 Invasive Hydatidiform Mole (Chorioadenoma Destruens) (Fig. 73)

A hydatidiform mole characterized by the presence of molar villi within the myometrium or its vessels.

The villi in an invasive mole are typically enlarged but often not to the same extent as in an intracavitary complete mole. Trophoblastic hyperplasia is variable. Even though myometrial or vascular invasion may not be demonstrated because the uterus is not available for pathologic examination, the presence of molar villi at an extrauterine site is presumptive evidence that the mole is invasive. In extrauterine sites the lesion is usually characterized by the presence of molar villi within blood vessels without invasion of adjacent tissue. In some cases, however, the lesion consists of a central hemorrhagic zone with surrounding molar villi and fibrosis. The diagnosis of an invasive mole cannot be made on examination of curettings except rarely, when curetted fragments of myometrium contain invasive molar villi.

3 Choriocarcinoma (Figs. 74–77)

An invasive neoplasm composed of trophoblast displaying a dimorphic pattern and lacking chorionic villi.

Choriocarcinoma may develop during or after any type of pregnancy. It is characterized by masses of cells invading adjacent tissue and permeating vascular spaces. Generally, it grows in an expansile, centrifugal fashion, usually accompanied by extensive hemorrhage and necrosis. Viable tumour may be limited to the interface of the tumour with the myometrium, forming a thin rim around a central area of hemorrhage and necrosis. Vascular invasion may be prominent since choriocarcinoma has no intrinsic vascular stroma. The growth pattern typically recapitulates that of previllous trophoblast, but other patterns may occur. All types of trophoblastic cells are present in varying proportions but in most cases there are areas in the tumour in which a clear-cut dimorphic pattern of cytotrophoblast and syncytiotrophoblast or of intermediate trophoblast and syncytiotrophoblast is present.

The presence of avillous trophoblast in curettings, especially small samples, may be very difficult to interpret. A number of points should be emphasized. The tendency of choriocarcinoma to undergo hemorrhage and necrosis may obscure its diagnostic features. On the other hand, the trophoblast in normal early gestation may look ominous and suggest choriocarcinoma. For a curetting to be diagnostic of choriocarcinoma, all the criteria for the diagnosis, particularly the presence of invasion and the absence of villi, must be established. Very rarely, however, choriocarcinoma is found in association with an abortus with immature villi or a mature placenta.

Choriocarcinoma is almost always gestational in origin irrespective of the site at which the presenting symptoms occur. Rarely, however, it has a gonadal or extragonadal nongestational origin, occurring either as a pure germ cell tumour or as a component of a mixed germ cell tumour. Tumours of nongestational origin have the same appearance as gestational choriocarcinomas; they are considered in more detail in the ovarian and testicular tumour classifications.

Nongestational choriocarcinomas also arise rarely from the somatic cells of a carcinoma. Such tumours usually display mixed patterns, with portions resembling the typical carcinoma of the organ or tissue involved and other portions having the appearance of choriocarcinoma. These tumours have been reported in the gastrointestinal tract, urinary bladder, breast, liver, lung, and uterus. In addition, tumours without the morphologic features of choriocarcinoma may produce various trophoblastic proteins such as chorionic gonadotropin (hCG) and placental lactogen (hPL).

4 Placental Site Trophoblastic Tumour (Figs. 78–82)

A trophoblastic tumour that forms a variably cellular mass occupying the endometrium and myometrium and resembling in its cellular composition nonneoplastic trophoblastic infiltration of the implantation site.

The predominant cellular population is intermediate trophoblast; cytotrophoblast and syncytiotrophoblast are relatively minor constituents. Most of the intermediate trophoblastic cells are mononucleate, but binucleate and multinucleate cells are usually present as well. There is a distinctive pattern of invasion, with the cells at the periphery of the tumour typically infiltrating singly or in small groups and dissecting between muscle fibers and bundles, without producing extensive necrosis in most of the cases. Highly cellular tumours, however, form solid masses and destroy the endometrium and myometrium. This tumour also exhibits a distinctive pattern of vascular invasion, characterized by mononucleate intermediate trophoblastic cells migrating through and replacing the walls of arteries. The presence of fibrinoid change in blood vessel walls is another characteristic feature.

In most cases the placental site trophoblastic tumour is benign, but occasionally it is highly malignant. Criteria to distinguish benign from malignant tumours have not been completely established; additionally, curettage may not yield tissue representative of the entire neoplasm. Increased mitotic activity is not a consistently reliable prognostic feature. Although most tumours with a mitotic count of less than 5 per 10 high power fields (HPF) in the most active areas have been benign, several fatal cases with mitotic counts under 5 per 10 HPF have been reported. Ominous features in several cases have been a preponderance of cells with clear rather than amphophilic cytoplasm, extensive necrosis, and hemorrhage.

When this tumour is clinically malignant it usually does not respond to chemotherapy as well as other forms of gestational trophoblastic disease. Serum hCG levels may not accurately reflect the extent of the disease since the placental site trophoblastic tumour may secrete only small quantities of hCG, even when widely disseminated.

5 Miscellaneous Trophoblastic Lesions

5.1 Exaggerated Placental Site (Figs. 83, 84)

An exuberant nonneoplastic proliferation of intermediate trophoblast at the implantation site.

This lesion may occur in association with normal pregnancy, an abortion, or a hydatidiform mole. On examination of curettings distinction from a placental site trophoblastic tumour may be difficult. If the process is focal, lacks mitotic activity, shows extensive hyalinization, and is admixed with fragments of decidua and chorionic villi, it is likely to be an exaggerated placental site. Invasion of spiral arteries by intermediate trophoblast normally occurs at the placental site and should not be considered evidence for a neoplasm. In contrast, a lesion with some features of an exaggerated placental site but composed of confluent masses of trophoblast or containing more than a rare mitotic figure should be classified as a placental site trophoblastic tumour. Villi are usually not identified in such cases.

5.2 Placental Site Nodule and Plaque (Figs. 85, 86)

One or more discrete nodules or plaques composed of intermediate tro-phoblastic cells embedded in hyalinized material.

Occasionally intermediate trophoblast is found in the form of one or more discrete nodules in the endometrium and superficial myometrium or in a plaque covering a variable extent of endometrium. The cells have little or no mitotic activity.

6 Unclassified Trophoblastic Lesions

Trophoblastic lesions not fulfilling the diagnostic criteria for a specific form of trophoblastic disease.

Included in this category are lesions with gross features of a mole but lacking abnormal trophoblastic activity and lesions displaying abnormal trophoblastic proliferation in association with nonmolar villi or without a villous component. The latter lesions lack the typical appearance of choriocarcinoma or placental site trophoblastic tumour. They should be described accurately and not classified specifically until their significance has been determined.

At times curettings obtained from a patient in whom a previous diagnosis of hydatidiform mole has been made contain fragments of avillous trophoblast with or without delineation into cytotrophoblast and syncytiotrophoblast or an admixture of intermediate trophoblast and blood clot. In such cases a diagnosis of persistent trophoblastic disease is appropriate. If the curettage followed a normal pregnancy or an abortion instead of a mole, diagnosis of "trophoblast suspicious for but not diagnostic of choriocarcinoma" may be rendered. Careful clinical follow-up with serum hCG assays should resolve the problem.

Trophoblastic cells, either alone or accompanied by villi, are occasionally deported to extrauterine sites, typically the lungs, vagina, or pelvic wall. The trophoblastic cells are predominantly of the intermediate type and the resultant lesion may closely simulate an exaggerated placental site. Although villous deportation occurs almost exclusively in association with an invasive complete hydatidiform mole, rarely, nonmolar villi are deported. These extrauterine lesions typically regress.

Uterine Cervix

1 Epithelial Tumours and Related Lesions

1.1 Squamous Lesions

1.1.1 Squamous Papilloma (Fig. 87)

A benign papillary tumour in which squamous epithelium without atypia lines a fibrovascular stalk.

The squamous papilloma is usually solitary, arising on the ectocervix or at the squamocolumnar junction. Evidence of human papilloma virus (HPV) infection is lacking. Squamous papillomas that contain a large amount of fibrous tissue in their stalks are sometimes referred to as "fibroepithelial polyps".

1.1.2 Condyloma Acuminatum (see Vulva, Figs. 165, 166)

A benign neoplasm characterized by papillary fronds containing fibrovascular cores and lined by stratified squamous epithelium with evidence of HPV infection, usually in the form of koilocytosis.

The typical condyloma acuminatum is relatively rare on the cervix. A more common manifestation of HPV infection of the cervix is a flat lesion with evidence of HPV infection. This lesion has been termed "flat condyloma" and "atypical condyloma" but is now classified within the spectrum of squamous intraepithelial lesions (dysplasia-carcinoma in situ; cervical intraepithelial neoplasia (CIN)).

1.1.3 Squamous Metaplasia (Fig. 88)

Replacement of endocervical epithelium by squamous epithelium, forming the transformation zone of the cervix.

The process is characterized in its early stages by proliferation of subcolumnar reserve cells, which gradually transform into mature squamous epithelium indistinguishable from the native squamous epithelium of the ectocervix. The terms "subcolumnar squamous metaplasia" and "immature squamous metaplasia" have been applied to the intermediate stages of the process. Squamous metaplasia must be distinguished from intraepithelial neoplasia. The cellular organization and the absence of nuclear atypia and atypical mitotic figures in metaplastic squamous epithelium are useful criteria in the differential dignosis. Squamous metaplasia involves both the surface columnar epithelium and endocervical glands.

1.1.4 Transitional Metaplasia (Fig. 89)

A transformation of native squamous epithelium or glandular epithelium of the cervix into transitional epithelium resembling that of the urinary tract.

The epithelium is characterized by cells with relatively clear cytoplasm and nuclei that typically contain grooves. Occasionally, when the cytoplasm of the cells is scanty and the nuclei are closely packed, transitional metaplasia resembles severe dysplasia – carcinoma in situ, but unlike the latter the transitional epithelium does not show nuclear variation, hyperchromatism, or mitotic activity.

1.1.5 Squamous Atypia (Fig. 90)

A squamous change characterized by uniform enlargement of nuclei, which typically contain prominent nucleoli.

This lesion may be associated with inflammation and regeneration or repair. A subset of cases of squamous atypia may be caused by HPV. The absence of more than minimal nuclear atypicality and the presence of prominent nucleoli are helpful in differentiating this lesion from dysplasia-carcinoma in situ.

1.1.6 Squamous Intraepithelial Lesions[1] (Dysplasia-Carcinoma In Situ; Cervical Intraepithelial Neoplasia (CIN)) (Figs. 91–95)

Squamous epithelial lesions characterized by disordered maturation and nuclear abnormalities such as loss of polarity, pleomorphism, coarsening of nuclear chromatin, irregularities of the nuclear membrane, and mitotic figures, including atypical forms, at various levels in the epithelium.

These lesions have been subdivided into three or four grades depending upon their extent and severity. They typically occur in the trans-

---

[1] The Bethesda System has recently been adopted by several cytology and pathology organizations for the classification of cytologic specimens from the female genital tract. According to this system the terms "low grade squamous intraepithelial lesion" and "high grade squamous intraepithelial lesion" are used to encompass the spectrum of intraepithelial lesions otherwise classified as dysplasia-carcinoma in situ (CIN). Cellular changes characteristic of HPV, mild dysplasia, and combinations of both are classified as low grade squamous intraepithelial lesions, and moderate and severe dysplasia-carcinoma in situ (CIN2 and 3) are classified as high grade squamous intraepithelial lesions.

formation zone and usually involve endocervical glands and surface epithelium. A small minority of them begin in the ectocervical epithelium.

1.1.6.1 Mild Dysplasia (CIN1) Figs. 91, 92)

Dysplasia confined to the lowest third of the epithelium.

Koilocytosis (koilocytotic atypia) in the upper third of the epithelium without nuclear abnormalities in the lower third is now placed in the category of mild dysplasia. Koilocytosis must be identified unequivocally to warrant the diagnosis of dysplasia. Enlarged, hyperchromatic, wrinkled nuclei must be present in the large cells with clear cytoplasm and thick cell membranes; the presence of binucleated or multinucleated clear cells provides additional evidence for the diagnosis. "Koilocytosis" and "koilocytotic atypia" are descriptive and not diagnostic terms; their presence may be mentioned in a note.

1.1.6.2 Moderate Dysplasia (CIN2) (Fig. 93)

Dysplasia involving the lower two thirds of the epithelium.

Some investigators include under moderate dysplasia those lesions in which nuclear abnormalities confined to the lower third of the epithelium are unusually severe.

1.1.6.3 Severe Dysplasia (CIN3) (Fig. 94)

Dysplasia extending into the upper third of the epithelium, but not involving the full thickness.

Some investigators include in the category of severe dysplasia those lesions in which the nuclear abnormalities in the lower and middle thirds are unusually severe.

1.1.6.4 Carcinoma In Situ (CIN3) (Fig. 95)

A squamous intraepithelial lesion in which nuclear abnormalities involve the full thickness of the epithelium.

A layer of keratin or a thin layer of desiccated cells on the surface does not exclude the diagnosis of carcinoma in situ.

1.1.7 Squamous Cell Carcinoma[2] (Figs. 96–103)

A carcinoma composed exclusively or almost exlusively of squamous cells.

Occasional tumour cells containing mucin may be demonstrated by special staining.

---

[2] Two major sets of criteria exist for the separation of microinvasive squamous cell carcinoma from more deeply invasive tumours (Figs. 96–98). The criteria set forth by

1.1.7.1 Keratinizing (Fig. 99)

A squamous cell carcinoma containing keratin pearls.

1.1.7.2 Nonkeratinizing (Figs. 100–102)

A squamous cell carcinoma that may contain individually keratinized cells but lacks keratin pearls.

The nonkeratinizing squamous cell carcinoma is the most frequent subtype of squamous cell carcinoma of the cervix. The cells are generally polygonal and less pleomorphic than those of the keratinizing squamous cell carcinoma. In some cases the tumour is composed of cells with abundant clear cytoplasm and must be distinguished from clear cell adenocarcinoma with a solid pattern. Some small cell carcinomas that show evidence of individual cell keratinization at a light microscopic level are included in the nonkeratinizing squamous cell category (Figs. 101, 102) and must be differentiated from the cervical small cell carcinoma that resembles small cell carcinoma of the lung.

1.1.7.3 Verrucous (see Vulva, Figs. 174, 175)

A highly differentiated squamous cell carcinoma that has a hyperkeratinized, undulating, warty surface and invades the underlying stroma in the form of bulbous pegs with a pushing border.

The tumour cells contain abundant cytoplasm, and their nuclei show no more than minimal atypicality. The lesion must be distinguished from condyloma acuminatum, which has sharper papillae with fibrovascular cores and typically pointed rather than broad projections into the underlying stroma; HPV changes are usually evident in condyloma acuminatum but not in verrucous carcinoma even though the latter has been shown to contain HPV in a few cases. It is important not to include in the verrucous carcinoma category squamous cell carcinomas that show more than minimal nuclear atypicality. Correctly diagnosed verrucous carcinomas have a tendency to recur locally after excision but do not metastasize.

1.1.7.4 Warty (Condylomatous) (see Vulva, Figs. 176, 177)

A squamous cell carcinoma with a warty surface and cellular features of HPV infection.

---

the International Federation of Gynecology and Obstetrics are: a depth below the surface epithelial basement membrane or the basement membrane of a glandular site of origin of 0.5 cm or less and a horizontal extent of 0.7 cm or less. Vascular space invasion is noted, if present, but does not in itself exclude a tumour from being placed in the microinvasive category. The Society of Gynecologic Oncologists (USA) requires that a microinvasive squamous cell carcinoma have a depth of invasion of 0.3 cm or less and show no vascular space invasion.

1.1.7.5 Papillary

A squamous cell carcinoma with a papillary architecture and a moderately or severely atypical squamous epithelial component.

This tumour is usually associated with invasion in the papillary stalks or the underlying cervical wall, but occasional tumours of this type have been entirely in situ. The presence of invasion must be excluded in cases in which a superficial biopsy specimen shows only in situ involvement.

1.1.7.6 Lymphoepithelioma-like Carcinoma (Fig. 103)

A carcinoma closely resembling a lymphoepithelial carcinoma of the nasopharynx, characterized by large undifferentiated neoplastic epithelial cells with abundant cytoplasm and a marked lymphoid infiltration of the stroma.

This tumour is usually well circumscribed and appears to have a better prognosis than typical squamous cell carcinoma.

1.2 Glandular Lesions

1.2.1 Endocervical Polyp (Fig. 104)

An intraluminal protrusion composed of endocervical glands and fibrous stroma.

The polyp may show a variety of alterations including inflammation, squamous metaplasia, squamous atypia, and dysplasia – carcinoma in situ.

1.2.2 Mullerian Papilloma (Fig. 105)

A unifocal or multifocal papillary lesion in which mullerian type columnar epithelium, which may undergo squamous metaplasia, lines thin fibrovascular stalks.

Inflammatory cell infiltration of the stroma is common.

1.2.3 Glandular Atypia

An atypical glandular epithelial alteration that does not fulfill the criteria for glandular dysplasia-adenocarcinoma in situ; it may be associated with inflammation.

1.2.4 Glandular Dysplasia (Fig. 106)

A glandular lesion characterized by significant nuclear abnormalities that are more striking than those encountered in glandular atypia but do not fulfill the criteria for adenocarcinoma in situ.

1.2.5 Adenocarcinoma In Situ (Figs. 107, 108)

A lesion in which normally situated glands are lined by cytologically malignant glandular epithelium.

The epithelial lining of the glands is usually devoid of intracellular mucin and may resemble endometrial epithelium; in some cases the glands are lined by intestinal type epithelium containing goblet cells and even argyrophil cells. The glands of adenocarcinoma in situ conform to the expected location of normal endocervical glands and do not extend deeper than the latter, do not have a complex pattern, and do not excite a desmoplastic stromal reaction. The lesion is commonly associated with squamous carcinoma in situ.

1.2.6 Adenocarcinoma

1.2.6.1 Mucinous Adenocarcinoma

An adenocarcinoma in which at least some of the cells contain a moderate to large amount of intracytoplasmic mucin.

1.2.6.1.1 Endocervical Type (Figs. 109–113)

A mucinous adenocarcinoma in which the mucinous cells resemble those of the endocervix.

Adenoma malignum (minimal deviation adenocarcinoma) is a generally highly differentiated mucinous adenocarcinoma in which most of the glands are impossible to distinguish histologically from normal endocervical glands (Figs. 110, 111); in the majority of cases, however, occasional glands have marked nuclear abnormalities or excite a desmoplastic stromal reaction or have both of these features. The tumour is more highly malignant than most varieties of endocervical adenocarcinoma. Some authors extend the designation "adenoma malignum" to include highly differentiated cervical adenocarcinomas of other cell types.

Villoglandular papillary adenocarcinomas have a villoglandular pattern and epithelial cells that are generally moderately to well differentiated (Figs. 112, 113). These tumours may not invade the cervical wall; when they invade, they typically have a pushing border. They appear to be associated with a better prognosis than adenocarcinomas of the cervix with other patterns.

1.2.6.1.2 Intestinal Type (Fig. 114)

An adenocarcinoma that resembles adenocarcinoma of the intestine, with goblet cells and occasionally argyrophil cells.

A very rare form of mucinous adenocarcinoma of the cervix is a signet-ring cell carcinoma, which must be distinguished from a metastatic signet-ring cell carcinoma of gastric or other origin.

1.2.6.2 Endometrioid Adenocarcinoma (Fig. 115)

An adenocarcinoma that has the microscopic features of an endometrioid adenocarcinoma of the endometrium.

This tumour must be distinguished from an endometrioid carcinoma that has extended into the cervix and from a cervical, poorly differentiated, mucinous adenocarcinoma that has few cells containing intracytoplasmic mucin. The endometrioid adenocarcinoma tends to have more rounded nuclei and to show less nuclear stratification than the poorly differentiated endocervical type of mucinous adenocarcinoma. The endometrioid adenocarcinoma may be highly differentiated like the typical adenoma malignum; occasionally it has a villoglandular pattern or contains numerous cystic glands.

1.2.6.3 Clear Cell Adenocarcinoma (see Vagina, Figs. 148–150)

An adenocarcinoma composed mainly of clear cells or hobnail cells arranged in solid, tubulocystic, or papillary patterns or a combination of these patterns.

This tumour is histologically similar to clear cell carcinomas of the ovary, uterine corpus, and vagina. The clear cell adenocarcinoma of the cervix is increased in frequency in patients who have been exposed to diethylstilbestrol or related nonsteroidal estrogens in utero.

1.2.6.4 Serous Adenocarcinoma (see Corpus, Fig. 18)

An adenocarcinoma characterized by a complex pattern of papillae with cellular budding and the frequent presence of psammoma bodies.

This tumour is rare in the cervix.

1.2.6.5 Mesonephric Adenocarcinoma (Figs. 116, 117)

An adenocarcinoma arising from mesonephric remnants in a lateral wall of the cervix and characterized in well differentiated areas by small glands lined by mucin-free cuboidal epithelium and containing eosinophilic, hyaline secretion in their lumens or by large tubular glands resembling those of endometrioid adenocarcinoma.

This tumour must be distinguished from focal and diffuse hyperplasia of mesonephric remnants, which may be extensive. The mesonephric adenocarcinoma usually arises on a background of mesonephric hyperplasia. Poorly differentiated mesonephric adenocarcinomas may have a solid architecture.

1.3 Other Epithelial Tumours

1.3.1 Adenosquamous Carcinoma (Fig. 118)

A carcinoma composed of a mixture of malignant glandular and squamous epithelial elements.

The glandular elements are typically of endocervical type but may be of endometrioid type. More than a minor component of glandular cells is required to alter the diagnosis from squamous cell carcinoma to adenosquamous carcinoma. Mucin stains are frequently helpful in recognizing the glandular component of the tumour.

1.3.2 Glassy Cell Carcinoma (Fig. 119)

A poorly differentiated carcinoma characterized by cells with abundant, ground-glass cytoplasm, sharp cell borders in well fixed specimens, and nuclei with single prominent nucleoli: minor amounts of glandular and squamous differentiation may be present.

This tumour may be infiltrated by large numbers of eosinophils. It is regarded by some observers as a poorly differentiated adenosquamous carcinoma.

1.3.3 Adenoid Cystic Carcinoma (Figs. 120, 121)

An adenocarcinoma of the cervix that resembles adenoid cystic carcinoma of salivary gland origin but usually lacks the myoepithelial cell component of the latter.

This tumour is composed of small basaloid cells arranged in well circumscribed sheets and nests, which typically have a cribriform pattern, with the spaces containing hyaline material or mucin; a hyaline stroma may form cylinders separating rows of tumour cells.

1.3.4 Adenoid Basal Carcinoma (Figs. 122, 123)

A cervical carcinoma in which rounded, generally well differentiated nests of basaloid cells show focal gland formation; central squamous differentiation may be present as well.

This tumour is almost always a small incidental finding in a cervical specimen removed because of the presence of dysplasia-carcinoma in situ or microinvasive squamous cell carcinoma. Unless it is poorly differentiated the adenoid basal carcinoma has an excellent prognosis.

1.3.5 Carcinoid Tumour (Fig. 124)

A tumour resembling carcinoid tumours of the gastrointestinal tract and lung.

1.3.6 Small Cell Carcinoma (Figs. 125, 126)

A cervical carcinoma resembling the small cell carcinoma of the lung.

This tumour should be differentiated from the small cell nonkeratinizing squamous cell carcinoma. The former has neuroendocrine features and little or no squamous differentiation, which, if present, is usually recognized only on electron microscopic examination. The small cell carcinoma typically grows diffusely, whereas the small cell squamous cell carcinoma usually contains discrete nests of tumour cells and is often associated with squamous dysplasia or carcinoma in situ.

1.3.7 Undifferentiated Carcinoma

A carcinoma that is not of the small cell type and lacks evidence of glandular, squamous or other types of differentiation.

2 Mesenchymal Tumours

2.1 Leiomyoma (see Corpus, Figs. 25–31)

2.2 Leiomyosarcoma (see Corpus, Figs. 32, 33)

This tumour is the most common sarcoma of the cervix. Its microscopic features are similar to those of leiomyosarcoma of the corpus.

2.3 Endocervical Stromal Sarcoma (Fig. 127)

A sarcoma composed of small spindle cells lacking specific features.

2.4 Sarcoma Botryoides (Embryonal Rhabdomyosarcoma)
(see Vagina, Figs. 152–154)

A tumour composed of cells with small, round to oval to spindle-shaped nuclei, some of which show evidence of differentiation towards striated muscle cells.

This tumour typically has a gross appearance resembling a bunch of grapes. It is similar microscopically to the sarcoma botryoides of the vagina (see page 59); islands of cartilage are often present, however, in the cervical tumour.

2.5 Endometrioid Stromal Sarcoma (see Corpus, Figs. 22–24)

This tumour may arise from endometriosis of the cervix. It must be distinguished from stromal endometriosis of the cervix and endometrial stromal sarcoma that has extended downward from the uterine corpus.

2.6 Alveolar Soft-Part Sarcoma

A sarcoma characterized by solid and alveolar groups of large epithelial-like cells with granular, eosinophilic cytoplasm; most of the tumours contain intracytoplasmic PAS-positive, diastase-resistant, rod-shaped crystals.

2.7 Others

A wide variety of other mesenchymal tumours have been reported in small numbers.

3 Mixed Epithelial and Mesenchymal Tumours

3.1 Adenofibroma (Fig. 128)

A tumour composed of benign epithelium of mullerian type and a mature fibroblastic stroma.

This tumour is characterized by the presence of broad, relatively acellular fibrous polyps covered typically by a flat or columnar mucinous epithelium, which may undergo focal squamous metaplasia.

3.2 Adenomyoma

3.2.1 Atypical Polypoid Adenomyoma (Variant)
(see Corpus, Figs. 39, 40)

3.3 Adenosarcoma (see Corpus, Figs. 41, 42)

A tumour composed of benign or atypical epithelium of mullerian type and a malignant appearing stroma.

The stroma may have the appearance of a fibrosarcoma or, less often, endometrial stromal sarcoma and may contain heterologous elements. The mullerian epithelium is usually mucinous but may undergo focal squamous metaplasia.

3.4 Malignant Mesodermal Mixed Tumour
(Malignant Mullerian Mixed Tumour, Carcinosarcoma)
(see Corpus, Figs. 43–45)

A malignant tumour composed of both carcinoma and sarcoma.

Like its more common counterpart in the corpus, the cervical tumour often contains heterologous elements.

3.5 Wilms Tumour

A malignant tumour showing primitive glomerular and tubal differentiation, resembling the Wilms tumour of the kidney.

This tumour is very rare in the cervix.

4 Miscellaneous Tumours

4.1 Melanocytic Naevus

4.2 Blue Naevus (Fig. 129)

This rare lesion has been found in the lower endocervix and in endocervical polyps.

4.3 Malignant Melanoma (see Vulva, Figs. 193–195)

This tumour has variable microscopic features similar to those of cutaneous melanomas. It may or may not contain melanin pigment.

4.4 Lymphoma and Leukemia (see Vagina, Fig. 157)

Lymphomas may be primary or secondary. Primary lymphomas typically cause diffuse or multinodular enlargement of the cervix with little or no overlying epithelial alteration. Rarely, leukemia presents as a cervical tumour.

4.5 Tumours of Germ Cell Type

4.5.1 Yolk Sac Tumour (Endodermal Sinus Tumour)

4.5.2 Dermoid Cyst (Mature Cystic Teratoma)

5 Secondary Tumours

The tumour that most commonly spreads to the cervix is carcinoma of the endometrium, followed by carcinomas of the ovary, breast, stomach, and large intestine.

6 Tumour-like Lesions

6.1 Endocervical Glandular Hyperplasia (Fig. 130)

Various forms of endocervical glandular hyperplasia are differentiated from adenocarcinoma by their orderly arrangement and bland nuclear features.

6.2 Cysts

Cystic dilatation of an endocervical gland (nabothian cyst) or of a gland lined by another type of epithelium, such as tubal or endometrioid epithelium, in the cervical wall.

These cysts may be deep in the cervical wall and must be distinguished from cystic glands of various adenocarcinomas.

6.3 Tunnel Cluster (Figs. 131, 132)

A well circumscribed, rounded aggregate of endocervical glands, which are usually dilated and lined by flat epithelium.

In its early stages the lesion may contain small closely packed glands.

6.4 Microglandular Hyperplasia (Figs. 133, 134)

A proliferation of endocervical glandular epithelium lacking significant nuclear atypicality, with the formation of small or occasionally cystically dilated glands containing mucin and frequently acute inflammatory cells.

This lesion occurs mostly in women who are pregnant or are receiving oral contraceptive therapy, but it may occur in a nonpregnant patient without known hormone ingestion. It must be differentiated from foci resembling it in cervical and endometrial adenocarcinomas.

6.5 Arias-Stella Change (Figs. 135, 136)

A transformation of endocervical glandular epithelial cells into hobnail cells with nuclear enlargement and hyperchromatism, occurring mainly during pregnancy.

This lesion is similar to that occurring in the endometrium during pregnancy or occasionally in association with hormone therapy. It must be distinguished from clear cell adenocarcinoma; mitotic activity is rare in the Arias-Stella change and the architectural features and invasiveness of clear cell adenocarcinoma are absent.

6.6 Mesonephric Remnants (Fig. 137)

Small tubules and ducts in the lateral walls of the cervix representing remnants of the mesonephric (wolffian) duct.

These structures have been found in 20%–25% of cervical specimens. The tubules are typically small and round, have a prominent basement membrane and contain dense, hyaline, eosinophilic secretion in their lumens.

6.7 Mesonephric Hyperplasia (Figs. 138–140)

An increase in the number of mesonephric ducts or tubules or both.

The tubular proliferation may be lobular or diffuse, with the tubules often infiltrating deeply and extensively into the cervical wall. Papillary hyperplasia may also occur within mesonephric ducts. Diffuse mesonephric hyperplasia must be distinguished from mesonephric adenocarcinoma, which is characterized by tubular crowding and significant nuclear atypicality.

6.8 Ciliated Cell Metaplasia (Fig. 141)

The presence of glands lined by ciliated cells; occasionally other tubal type epithelial cells are present as well.

This lesion is common, with the affected glands often situated more deeply in the cervical wall than the normal endocervical glands.

6.9 Intestinal Metaplasia

A change of endocervical epithelium into epithelium containing goblet cells and occasionally argentaffin and Paneth cells.

6.10 Epidermal metaplasia

The appearance of keratinized epithelium resembling epidermis, rarely accompanied by sebaceous glands and hair follicles.

6.11 Endometriosis (Fig. 142)

The presence of endometrial-type glands and stroma or stroma alone in the cervix, usually on the portio.

Pure stromal endometriosis has to be distinguished from low grade endometrial stromal sarcoma.

6.12 Ectopic Decidua (Fig. 143)

Enlargement of stromal cells with acquisition of abundant cytoplasm resembling decidual cells of the endometrium.

6.13 Placental Site Nodule and Plaque
(see Gestational Trophoblastic Disease, Figs. 85, 86)

One or more discrete nodules or plaques composed of intermediate trophoblastic cells embedded in hyalinized material.

The lesion is sometimes confused with microinvasive squamous cell carcinoma.

6.14 Stromal Polyp (Pseudosarcoma Botryoides)
(see Vagina, Figs. 158, 159)

A polyp composed of hypocellular stroma containing small spindle cells and large, stellate cells with multiple tapering processes.

This benign lesion is differentiated from sarcoma botryoides by its usual rarity of mitotic figures, absence of rhabdomyoblasts, and absence of a cambium layer.

6.15 Postoperative Spindle Cell Nodule
(see Vagina, Figs. 160, 161)

A localized benign lesion composed of closely packed proliferating spindle cells and capillaries occurring several weeks to several months postoperatively in the region of an incision.

This lesion may resemble closely a leiomyosarcoma but the circumstance of its origin facilitates its diagnosis.

6.16 Traumatic (Amputation) Neuroma

A proliferation of nerves following a surgical operation on the cervix.

6.17 Retention of Fetal Glial Tissue

A polypoid mass composed of glial tissue, which typically follows an incomplete abortion.

6.18 Lymphoma-like Lesions (see Corpus, Fig. 62)

Nonneoplastic proliferations of lymphoid tissue that resemble malignant lymphoma.

Unlike lymphomas, lymphoma-like lesions are typically small, extend to the surface epithelium, do not infiltrate deeply, do not form collars around blood vessels, and contain a variety of inflammatory cells types. Occasional examples are a manifestation of infectious mononucleosis.

Vagina

1 Epithelial Tumours and Related Lesions

1.1 Squamous Lesions

1.1.1 Squamous Papilloma (see Cervix, Fig. 87; Vulva, Fig. 163)

A benign papillary tumour in which squamous epithelium without atypia lines a fibrovascular stalk.

This lesion is usually multiple, occurring anywhere in the vagina but typically around the hymenal ring, where there may be continuity with similar lesions in the vulvar vestibule. The lesions lack the cytologic features of HPV infection.

1.1.2 Condyloma Acuminatum (see Vulva, Figs. 165, 166)

A benign neoplasm characterized by papillary fronds containing fibro-vascular cores and lined by stratified squamous epithelium with evidence of HPV infection, usually in the form of koilocytosis.

1.1.3 Transitional Metaplasia (see Cervix, Fig. 89)

A transformation of native squamous epithelium into transitional epithelium resembling that of the urinary tract.

The epithelium is composed of cells with relatively clear cytoplasm and pale nuclei that typically contain grooves. Occasionally, when the nuclei are closely packed this lesion resembles severe dysplasia-carcinoma in situ, but nuclear variation, hyperchromatism and mitotic activity are absent.

1.1.4 Squamous Atypia (see Cervix, Fig. 90)

A squamous change characterized by uniform enlargement of nuclei, which typically contain prominent nucleoli.

This lesion may be accompanied by inflammatory cell infiltration of the underlying stroma.

1.1.5 Squamous Intraepithelial Lesions[3]
(Dysplasia – Carcinoma In Situ; Vaginal Intraepithelial
Neoplasia (VAIN)) (see Cervix, Figs. 91–95)

1.1.5.1 Mild Dysplasia (VAIN1) (see Cervix, Figs. 91, 92)

1.1.5.2 Moderate Dysplasia (VAIN2) (see Cervix, Fig. 93)

1.1.5.3 Severe Dysplasia (VAIN3) (see Cervix, Fig. 94)

1.1.5.4 Carcinoma In Situ (VAIN3) (see Cervix, Fig. 95)

Criteria for diagnosing the above lesions of the vagina are similar to those used in the diagnosis of corresponding cervical lesions. Vaginal dysplasia-carcinoma in situ may follow radiation therapy. In most cases the lesion develops from the native squamous epithelium but it may also develop in women with adenosis in a manner similar to the development of dysplasia-carcinoma in situ in the transformation zone of the cervix.

1.1.6 Squamous Cell Carcinoma (see Cervix, Figs. 96–102)

1.1.6.1 Keratinizing (see Cervix, Fig. 99)

1.1.6.2 Nonkeratinizing (see Cervix, Figs. 100–102)

1.1.6.3 Verrucous (see Vulva, Figs. 174, 175)

1.1.6.4 Warty (Condylomatous) (see Vulva, Figs. 176, 177)

Squamous cell carcinoma of the vagina must be distinguished from the more common secondary squamous cell carcinomas that have extended into the vagina from the cervix or the vulva. If a tumour involves both the vagina and the cervix, it is considered to be primary in the cervix in most cases. Also, a history of a previous in situ or invasive cervical or vulvar carcinoma within 5–10 years before the appearance of the vaginal tumour is considered to exclude the diagnosis of primary vaginal carcinoma in most cases.

---

[3] The Bethesda System has recently been adopted by several cytology and pathology organizations for the classification of cytologic specimens from the female genital tract. According to this system the terms "low grade squamous intraepithelial lesion" and "high grade squamous intraepithelial lesion" are used to encompass the spectrum of intraepithelial lesions otherwise classified as dysplasia-carcinoma in situ (VAIN). Cellular changes characteristic of HPV, mild dysplasia, and combinations of both are classified as low grade squamous intraepithelial lesions, and moderate and severe dysplasia-carcinoma in situ (VAIN2 and 3) are classified as high grade squamous intraepithelial lesions.

1.2 Glandular Lesions

1.2.1 Mullerian Papilloma (see Cervix, Fig. 105)

A unifocal or multifocal papillary lesion in which mullerian type epithelium, which may undergo squamous metaplasia, lines thin fibrovascular stalks.

This lesion has been reported most frequently in infants and young children.

1.2.2 Adenosis (Figs. 144–147)

The presence of glandular epithelium or its secretory products in the vagina.

The presence of glandular epithelium in the vagina in very small amounts is relatively common, as demonstrated by extensive sectioning at autopsy. Clinically significant vaginal adenosis, however, is relatively uncommon and has been encountered most often in young females who had been exposed in utero to diethylstilbestrol or chemically related nonsteroidal estrogens. The process has also been seen above an imperforate hymen and after laser therapy or treatment with 5-fluorouracil. Although the term "adenosis" applies to the presence of glands or cysts lined by any type of glandular epithelium, the clinically significant forms of adenosis are characterized by an endocervical or a tuboendometrial type of epithelium, which may be ciliated. The endocervical type epithelium may lie on the surface or line glands, and the tuboendometrial type of epithelium typically lines glands in the lamina propria. Vaginal adenosis due to prenatal hormone exposure may disappear as a result of squamous metaplasia, with complete maturation and reconstitution of the architecture of the vaginal wall. In the later phases of healing of vaginal adenosis the only evidence of its previous presence may be the identification of small pools of mucin or intracellular droplets of mucin within squamous cells.

1.2.3 Atypical Adenosis

Adenosis in which the glandular epithelium shows varying degrees of nuclear pleomorphism, hyperchromatism, and nucleolar prominence.

Atypicality has been reported in the tuboendometrial form of adenosis and may be a precursor of clear cell adenocarcinoma.

1.2.4 Adenocarcinoma

1.2.4.1 Clear Cell Adenocarcinoma (Figs. 148–150)

An adenocarcinoma composed mainly of clear cells or hobnail cells, arranged in solid, tubulocystic, or papillary patterns, or a combination of these patterns.

Clear cell adenocarcinoma has been encountered most often in association with the vaginal adenosis that complicates prenatal exposure to diethylstilbestrol and related drugs. In almost all the cases in this category the carcinoma lies adjacent to areas of vaginal adenosis, characteristically of the tuboendometrial type. The most common site of the carcinoma is the anterior wall of the upper third of the vagina.

1.2.4.2 Endometrioid Adenocarcinoma (see Cervix, Fig. 115)

1.2.4.3 Mucinous Adenocarcinoma

1.2.4.3.1 Endocervical Type (see Cervix, Figs. 109–113)

1.2.4.3.2 Intestinal Type (see Cervix, Fig. 114)

The above three varieties of vaginal adenocarcinoma are rare and resemble tumours of similar types encountered more commonly in the endometrium, cervix and intestine, respectively.

1.2.4.4 Mesonephric Adenocarcinoma (see Cervix, Figs. 116, 117)

1.3 Other Epithelial Tumours

1.3.1 Adenosquamous Carcinoma (see Cervix, Fig. 118)

1.3.2 Adenoid Cystic Carcinoma (see Cervix, Figs. 120, 121)

1.3.3 Adenoid Basal Carcinoma (see Cervix, Figs. 122, 123)

1.3.4 Carcinoid Tumour (see Cervix, Fig. 124)

1.3.5 Small Cell Carcinoma (see Cervix, Figs. 125, 126)

1.3.6 Undifferentiated Carcinoma

All of these tumours are very rare and are similar microscopically to those occurring in the cervix.

2 Mesenchymal Tumours

2.1 Leiomyoma (see Corpus, Figs. 25–29)

Leiomyomas are the most common mesenchymal tumour of the vagina of adults.

2.2 Rhabdomyoma (Fig. 151)

Rhabdomyomas form solid, nodular, or polypoid masses and are composed of mature striated muscle cells separated by varying amounts of fibrous stroma. Unlike the embryonal rhabdomyosarcoma, the rhabdomyoma has been reported in the vagina of adult patients.

2.3 Leiomyosarcoma (see Corpus, Figs. 32, 33)

Leiomyosarcoma is the most common malignant mesenchymal tumour of the vagina of adults.

2.4 Sarcoma Botryoides (Embryonal Rhabdomyosarcoma) (Figs. 152–154)

A tumour composed of cells with small round to oval to spindle-shaped nuclei, some of which show evidence of differentiation towards striated muscle cells.

The tumour typically presents as a multipolypoid mass resembling a bunch of grapes. The vaginal sarcoma botryoides occurs almost exclusively in infants and young children. The tumour characteristically contains a cambium layer of closely packed cells with small hyperchromatic nuclei lying immediately beneath the squamous epithelium; occasionally tumour cells invade the epithelium. The central portions of the polypoid masses are typically hypocellular and edematous or myxomatous.

2.5 Endometrioid Stromal Sarcoma (see Corpus, Figs. 22–24)

This tumour, which has microscopic features similar to those of the uterine tumour of the same type, may be primary, occasionally arising in endometriosis, but metastatic sarcoma from the uterus must be excluded before making the diagnosis.

2.6 Others

A variety of other benign and malignant mesenchymal tumours occur rarely in the vagina.

3 Mixed Epithelial and Mesenchymal Tumours

3.1 Mixed Tumour (Figs. 155, 156)

A generally benign, well circumscribed tumour composed mainly of mesenchymal appearing cells and to a lesser extent of epithelial cells of either squamous or mucinous type.

This tumour typically occurs just above the hymen.

3.2 Adenosarcoma (see Corpus, Figs. 41, 42)

3.3 Malignant Mesodermal Mixed Tumour
(Malignant Mullerian Mixed Tumour; Carcinosarcoma)
(see Corpus, Figs. 43–45)

This tumour arises rarely in the vagina; extension from elsewhere in the female genital tract must be excluded before making the diagnosis.

3.4 Mixed Tumour Resembling Synovial Sarcoma

A very rare malignant tumour with a biphasic pattern containing gland-like structures lined by flat cells with an epithelial appearance and resembling synovial sarcoma.

4 Miscellaneous Tumours

4.1 Melanocytic Naevus

4.2 Blue Naevus (see Cervix, Fig. 129)

These lesions are very rare in the vagina.

4.3 Malignant Melanoma (see Vulva, Figs. 193–195)

Vaginal malignant melanomas may be pigmented or amelanotic. Their microscopic features resemble those of malignant melanoma elsewhere.

4.4 Tumours of Germ Cell Type

4.4.1 Yolk Sac Tumour (Endodermal Sinus Tumour)

The yolk sac tumour is the most common form of germ cell tumour in the vagina, which is the most frequent site of this tumour in the lower genital tract. The tumour occurs typically in young children and is composed of primitive epithelial cells typically arranged in a microcystic or reticular pattern; Schiller-Duval bodies and intracellular hyaline globules are characteristic features. Alpha-fetoprotein is almost always demonstrable in the tumour.

4.4.2 Dermoid Cyst (Mature Cystic Teratoma)

4.5 Adenomatoid Tumour (see Corpus, Figs. 37, 38)

This tumour is very rare in the vagina.

4.6 Villous Adenoma

A tumour resembling a villous adenoma of the large intestine.

4.7 Lymphoma and Leukemia (Fig. 157)

These tumours rarely originate in the vagina; more often their presence in the vagina is a manifestation of generalized disease.

5 Secondary Tumours

These tumours are more common than primary vaginal cancers. The primary tumour that spreads most often to the vagina is cervical carcinoma, followed by carcinoma of the vulva. Endometrial, intestinal, ovarian, urinary tract, and renal cancers and other malignant tumours also spread to the vagina.

6 Tumour-like Lesions

6.1 Stromal Polyp (Pseudosarcoma Botryoides)
(Figs. 158, 159)

A fibroepithelial polyp lined by squamous epithelium and containing a central core of fibrous tissue in which stellate cells with tapering cytoplasmic processes and irregularly shaped thin-walled vessels are prominent features.

This lesion can occur at any age but has a predilection for pregnant women. Because of the presence of nuclear atypicality the lesion must be distinguished from sarcoma botryoides, but a cambium layer and rhabdomyoblasts are absent and mitotic activity is typically low.

6.2 Postoperative Spindle Cell Nodule (Figs. 160, 161)

A localized, benign lesion composed of closely packed proliferating spindle cells and capillaries simulating a leiomyosarcoma and occurring several weeks to several months postoperatively in the region of an incision.

This lesion is mitotically active and may infiltrate underlying tissue. The distinction from a malignant spindle cell tumour depends to a large extent on history of a recent operation at the same site.

6.3 Vault Granulation Tissue

Granulation tissue, typically containing acute and chronic inflammatory cells and developing at the vaginal apex after hysterectomy.

6.4 Prolapse of Fallopian Tube (Fig. 162)

A polypoid mass at the vaginal apex composed of papillary fronds lined by fallopian tube epithelium, occurring after a hysterectomy, usually a vaginal hysterectomy.

This lesion must be distinguished from papillary adenocarcinoma, with which it is occasionally confused.

6.5 Endometriosis (see Cervix, Fig. 142)

6.6 Ectopic Decidua (see Cervix, Fig. 143)

This stromal alteration may occur in patients who are pregnant or are receiving progestin therapy.

6.7 Cysts

6.7.1 Epidermal

A cyst lined by squamous epithelium.
    This lesion may follow surgical trauma with implantation of squamous epithelium below the epithelial surface.

6.7.2 Mullerian

A cyst lined by endocervical, endometrial, or tubal type epithelium.

6.7.3 Mesonephric

A cyst lined by non-mucin-containing cuboidal epithelium located in a lateral wall of the vagina.

6.8 Microglandular Hyperplasia (see Cervix, Figs. 133, 134)

This lesion arises rarely in vaginal adenosis and must be differentiated from clear cell adenocarcinoma.

6.9 Lymphoma-like Lesions (see Corpus, Fig. 62)

Vulva

1 Epithelial Tumours and Related Lesions

1.1 Squamous Lesions

1.1.1 Epithelial Papillomas and Polyps

1.1.1.1 Vestibular Squamous Papilloma (Vestibular Papilloma) (Fig. 163)

A benign papillary tumour in which squamous epithelium without atypia lines a delicate fibrovascular stalk.

Evidence of HPV infection is lacking. The lesion may be single or multiple, often occurring as clusters of papillae less than 0.6 cm in height.

1.1.1.2 Fibroepithelial Polyp (Fig. 164)

A polypoid lesion, usually solitary, characterized by a prominent fibrovascular core covered by squamous epithelium that may be acanthotic and hyperkeratotic but lacks evidence of HPV infection.

1.1.2 Condyloma Acuminatum (Figs. 165, 166)

A benign neoplasm characterized by papillary fronds containing fibrovascular cores and lined by stratified squamous epithelium with evidence of HPV infection, usually in the form of koilocytosis (see Cervix, Fig. 92).

Lesions of this type are caused mostly by HPV 6, 11 and 16, although type 18 and some types in the 30s and 40s have also been identified. The lesion is typically multiple and papillomatous or papular. The epithelium is acanthotic with parabasal hyperplasia and koilocytosis in the upper portion; hyperkeratosis and parakeratosis are usual, and binucleated and multinucleated keratinocytes are often present. The rete ridges are elongated and thickened. A chronic inflammatory infiltrate is usually present within the underlying connective tissue.

HPV presence in the vulvar epithelium occurs in three broad categories: fully expressed, with numerous morphologic features of HPV infection, as seen in condyloma acuminatum; minimally expressed, with only slight morphologic changes, e. g., koilocytosis; and latent, in which no characteristic morphologic changes are seen, but HPV is found with the use of molecular biologic techniques.

1.1.3 Seborrheic Keratosis

A benign tumour characterized by proliferation of the basal cells of the squamous epithelium with acanthosis, hyperkeratosis, and the formation of keratin-filled "horn" cysts.

1.1.4 Keratoacanthoma

A benign squamous epithelial tumour with a central keratin-filled crater and focal infiltration at its dermal interface.

The growth of this tumour is self-limited and it typically regresses spontaneously.

1.1.5 Squamous Intraepithelial Lesions (Dysplasia-Carcinoma In Situ, Vulvar Intraepithelial Neoplasia (VIN))

Squamous epithelial lesions characterized by disordered maturation and nuclear abnormalities such as loss of polarity, pleomorphism, coarsening of nuclear chromatin, irregularities of the nuclear membrane and mitotic figures, including atypical forms, at various levels in the epithelium.

The epithelial cells are typically crowded, and acanthosis may be present. A prominent granular layer may be associated with parakeratosis, hyperkeratosis, or both. Involvement of skin appendages is seen in over one third of the cases. In hairy skin this involvement may be as deep as 2.7 mm whereas in nonhairy sites the depth of involvement is usually not greater than 1 mm. Skin appendage involvement should not be misinterpreted as invasive squamous cell carcinoma.

When HPV changes are associated with an intraepithelial lesion, a phrase such as "with", "with adjacent", or "with remote human papillomavirus changes", or "with condyloma acuminatum" should be added. When koilocytosis is seen without other diagnostic HPV changes, a phrase such as "with koilocytosis" may be added.

"Bowenoid papulosis" is unacceptable as a histopathologic diagnosis in the vulva. It is used by clinicians to describe distinctive clinical features, including spontaneous regression of a lesion that shows on biopsy the features of dysplasia-carcinoma in situ. A statement such as "the microscopic findings are consistent with the clinical diagnosis of bowenoid papulosis" can be added to the pathology report if appropriate.

Some squamous intraepithelial lesions, including mild dysplasia, are occasionally associated with invasive squamous cell carcinoma.

1.1.5.1 Mild Dysplasia (VIN1)

Dysplasia confined to the lowest third of the epithelium.

Koilocytosis, individual cell keratinization, and other features of HPV infection may be present; abnormal mitotic figures can usually be found but are generally rare. This lesion must not be confused with the simplex type of carcinoma in situ (see below).

1.1.5.2 Moderate Dysplasia (VIN2) (Fig. 167)

Dysplasia involving the lower two thirds of the epithelium.

1.1.5.3 Severe Dysplasia (VIN3) (Fig. 168)

Dysplasia extending into the upper third of the epithelium, but not involving the full thickness.

1.1.5.4 Carcinoma In Situ (VIN3) (Figs. 169, 170)

A squamous intraepithelial lesion in which nuclear abnormalities involve the full thickness of the epithelium or in which the lower portion of the epithelium is replaced by a lesion resembling grade 1 squamous cell carcinoma.

The presence of a granular layer, hyperkeratosis, or parakeratosis should not exclude the diagnosis of carcinoma in situ.

Severe dysplasia-carcinoma in situ encompasses the lesions that have been designated "Bowen disease" "erythroplasia of Queyrat" and "carcinoma in situ, simplex type" (Fig. 170). The last term has been used to characterize a highly differentiated lesion in which the atypia is most prominent in or confined to the basal and parabasal layers of the epithelium, where the cells have abundant cytoplasm and form pearls; the nuclei are relatively uniform in size and contain coarse chromatin and prominent nucleoli.

1.1.6 Squamous Cell Carcinoma (Figs. 171–179)

A carcinoma composed of squamous cells of varying degrees of differentiation.

Squamous cell carcinoma is the most common malignant tumour of the vulva, increasing in incidence with age. It is usually solitary and is found most commonly on the labia minora or majora; the clitoris is the primary site in approximately 10% of the cases.

1.1.6.1 Keratinizing (see Cervix, Fig. 99)

A squamous cell carcinoma containing keratin pearls.

1.1.6.2 Nonkeratinizing (Figs. 171, 172)

A squamous cell carcinoma that may contain small numbers of individually keratinized cells but lacks keratin pearls.

Rarely the tumour is composed predominantly of spindle cells.

1.1.6.3 Basaloid (Fig. 173)

A squamous cell carcinoma composed of nests of immature, basal type squamous cells with scanty cytoplasm, which resemble closely the cells of squamous carcinoma in situ of the cervix.

Keratinization may be evident in the centres of the nests, but keratin pearls are rarely present. This tumour may be associated with HPV infection, predominantly type 16.

1.1.6.4 Verrucous (Figs. 174, 175)

A highly differentiated squamous cell carcinoma that has a hyperkeratinized, undulating, warty surface and invades the underlying stroma in the form of bulbous pegs with a pushing border.

Verrucous carcinomas account for 1 %–2 % of all vulvar carcinomas and have little or no metastatic potential. The cellular features include minimal nuclear atypicality and abundant eosinophilic cytoplasm. Mitotic figures are rare and, when present, are typical. There is usually a prominent chronic inflammatory cell infiltrate in the stroma. HPV, especially type 6, has been identified in a number of cases. The giant condyloma of Buschke and Lowenstein is now considered to be verrucous carcinoma.

1.1.6.5 Warty (Condylomatous) (Figs. 176, 177)

A squamous cell carcinoma with a warty surface and cellular features of HPV infection.

This tumour may be associated with HPV infection, predominantly type 16.

1.1.6.6 Others

These include acantholytic squamous cell carcinomas, in which gland-like spaces result from acantholysis, and squamous cell carcinomas with a prominent giant cell component.

In 1984 the International Society for the Study of Vulvar Disease (ISSVD) proposed the term "stage Ia carcinoma", defining it as "a single lesion measuring 2 cm or less in diameter with a depth of invasion of 1 mm or less". Cases in which there is more than one site of invasion are not included in this category.[4] The use of the term "microinvasion" is not recommended. The depth of invasion (in millimeters) and the thickness of the tumour (in millimeters) should be reported.

The measurement from the epithelial-stromal junction of the most superficial adjacent dermal papilla to the deepest point of invasion is referred to as "the depth of invasion".[5] The measurement should be made with a calibrated ocular micrometer or other suitable measurement device (Figs. 178, 179).

Measurement from the tumour surface, or granular layer if keratinization is present, to the deepest point of invasion should be referred to as the "thickness" of the tumour. When a carcinoma in situ is above the invasive tumour, its thickness should be included in the measurement of the tumour thickness. The measurement should be made with a calibrated ocular micrometer or other suitable measurement device.[6]

The diameter of the tumour may be measured in the fresh or fixed state and should be confirmed histologically, with exclusion of adjacent vulvar intraepithelial neoplasia from the measurement. It should be stated whether the tumour has been measured in the fixed or fresh state.

It is recommended that the following information regarding the primary tumour be included in the final pathology report:
1. Depth of invasion
2. Thickness of the tumour
3. Methods of measurement of the depth of invasion and thickness
4. Diameter of the invasive tumour
5. Clinical measurement of the tumour diameter, when available
6. Presence or absence of vascular space involvement by tumour

1.1.7 Basal Cell Carcinoma (Fig. 180)

An infiltrating tumour composed predominantly of cells resembling the basal cells of the epidermis.

Squamous cell differentiation may occur at the center of the tumour nests. When gland-like structures are present the tumour is referred to as "adenoid basal cell carcinoma". When infiltrating squamous cells are

---

[4] International Society for the Study of Vulvar Disease (1984) Microinvasive cancer of the vulva: report of the ISSVD Task Force. J Reprod Med 29: 454–456.

[5] Wilkinson EJ, Rico MJ, Pierson KK (1982) Microinvasive carcinoma of the vulva. Int J Gynecol Pathol 1: 29–39.

[6] Dvoretsky P, Bonfiglio T, Helmkamp F, et al. (1984) The pathology of superficially invasive, thin vulvar squamous cell carcinoma. Int J Gynecol Pathol 3: 331–342.

also present the terms "metatypical basal cell carcinoma" and "baso-squamous carcinoma" have been used.

1.2 Glandular Lesions

1.2.1 Papillary Hidradenoma (Figs. 181–183)

A benign tumour of eccrine sweat gland origin composed of epithelial se-cretory cells and underlying myoepithelial cells lining complex branching papillae with delicate fibrovascular stalks.

This tumour is the most common benign glandular neoplasm of the vulva; all other forms are rare. The tumour location ranges from the lateral aspect of the labium minus to the lateral aspect of the labium majus.

1.2.2 Clear Cell Hidradenoma

1.2.3 Syringoma

1.2.4 Trichoepithelioma

1.2.5 Trichilemmoma

1.2.6 Adenoma of Minor Vestibular Glands

A benign tumour of the vestibule composed of clusters of small glands lined by mucin-secreting columnar epithelial cells.

This rare tumour is usually an incidental finding 1–2 mm in diameter.

1.2.7 Paget Disease (Figs. 184–186)

A carcinoma composed of glandular cells usually confined to the squa-mous epithelium, but accompanied by invasive adenocarcinoma in 10%–20% of the cases.

Paget cells typically lie within the squamous epithelium as single cells or clusters of cells with pale or vacuolated cytoplasm. The nuclei usually have prominent nucleoli and finely granular chromatin. The cells may be seen at all levels of the epithelium, including the granular and keratin layers. Unlike keratinocytes, Paget cells do not mature within the squamous epithelium. The cytoplasm of some of the cells contains neutral and acid mucopolysaccharides and carcinoembryonic antigen (CEA); stains for these substances are of use in distinguishing Paget cells from keratinocytes and melanocytes; Paget cells may contain melanin granules.

1.2.8 Bartholin Gland Carcinomas

Carcinomas of diverse types that are located at the site of the gland, have a microscopic appearance consistent with a Bartholin gland type of carcinoma, and are shown not to be metastatic from another site.

1.2.8.1 Adenocarcinoma (Fig. 187)

This tumour is typically composed of cells that contain mucin; it may be papillary. It accounts for 40 % of Bartholin gland tumours.

1.2.8.2 Squamous Cell Carcinoma

This tumour accounts for 40 % of Bartholin gland tumours.

1.2.8.3 Adenoid Cystic Carcinoma (see Cervix, Figs. 120, 121)

A carcinoma composed typically of rounded islands of uniform malignant epithelial cells with a cribriform pattern; a hyaline stroma may form cylinders separating rows of tumour cells.
    This tumour accounts for 15 % of Bartholin gland tumours.

1.2.8.4 Adenosquamous Carcinoma

A carcinoma composed of mucin-containing glandular cells and squamous cells.

1.2.8.5 Transitional Cell Carcinoma

A carcinoma composed of urothelial type cells, occasionally with a minor component of glandular or squamous cells.

1.2.9 Tumours Arising from Ectopic Breast Tissue

Carcinomas resembling breast carcinomas, mostly of the infiltrating ductal type, as well as a variety of benign and other malignant tumours of mammary type rarely arise in ectopic breast tissue.

1.2.10 Carcinomas of Sweat Gland Origin

These tumours include eccrine adenocarcinoma, porocarcinoma, hidradenocarcinoma, and apocrine adenocarcinoma, the last of which may be associated with Paget disease.

1.2.11 Adenocarcinomas of Other Types

These tumours may arise from Skene glands or ectopic cloacal tissue.

2 Soft Tissue Tumours

These are defined according to the WHO histological classification of soft tissue tumours.

2.1 Benign

2.1.1 Lipoma and Fibrolipoma

2.1.2 Haemangiomas

2.1.2.1 Capillary

The capillary haemangioma encountered in infants and young children typically regresses spontaneously.

2.1.2.2 Cavernous

This tumour may be associated with cavernous haemangiomas of the upper genital tract.

2.1.2.3 Acquired

Haemangiomas that develop in adults are composed of small thin-walled vessels lined by mature, flat endothelial cells; the vascular lumens tend to become dilated with advancing age. These tumours are seen most often in elderly women, presenting as multiple 1–3 mm papules on the lateral aspects of the labia majora.

2.1.3 Angiokeratoma

A tumour composed of dilated, thin-walled blood vessels in the upper dermis, associated with overlying epidermal hyperplasia and hyperkeratosis.

Angiokeratomas are common on the vulva during the reproductive years, occurring as solitary or multiple, warty or polypoid lesions.

2.1.4 Pyogenic Granuloma

2.1.5 Lymphangioma

Lymphangiomas are rare in the vulva, where they may be congenital or acquired. The congenital form may be accompanied by lymphangiomas of the lower extremities.

2.1.6 Fibroma

2.1.7 Leiomyoma (see Corpus, Figs. 25–29)

This tumour may show myxoid change, especially during pregnancy; occasional leiomyomas of the vulva are of the epithelioid type.

2.1.8 Granular Cell Tumour (Figs. 188, 189)

A tumour composed of cells with uniform central nuclei and abundant granular eosinophilic cytoplasm.

This tumour is thought to be derived from the Schwann cell and is positive for S-100 protein. Between 5% and 10% of granular cell tumours occur in the vulva. They are almost always benign and may be multiple. Often the tumour elicits hyperplasia of the overlying squamous epithelium, which may closely mimic squamous cell carcinoma.

2.1.9 Neurofibroma

A benign, usually unencapsulated tumour composed of Schwann cells and other nerve sheath cells, including perineurial fibroblasts; axons are frequently entrapped.

Almost half the neurofibromas of the vulva occur in association with von Recklinghausen neurofibromatosis.

2.1.10 Schwannoma (Neurilemoma)

A benign, encapsulated tumour composed of Schwann cells.

2.1.11 Glomus Tumour

2.1.12 Benign Fibrous Histiocytoma

This tumour has also been referred to as dermatofibroma, subepidermal nodular fibrosis, histiocytoma, and sclerosing haemangioma.

2.1.13 Rhabdomyoma

2.2 Malignant

2.2.1 Embryonal Rhabdomyosarcoma (Sarcoma Botryoides)
(see Vagina, Figs. 152–154)

When this tumour arises in the vulva it typically forms a solid mass instead of having a multipolypoid (botryoid) appearance.

2.2.2 Aggressive Angiomyxoma (Figs. 190, 191)

A locally invasive tumour composed of well differentiated spindle cells lying in a myxoid and collagenous stroma that contains blood vessels, which may be thick-walled.
   This rare tumour presents as a mass in the vulva or elsewhere in the perineal region; it often extends into the pelvis and has a strong tendency to recur if it has not been excised widely.

2.2.3 Leiomyosarcoma (see Corpus, Figs. 32, 33)

This tumour is the most common sarcoma of the vulva. When it is low grade it may be difficult to distinguish from a leiomyoma. The size of the tumour, the character of its margin, the degree of nuclear atypicality, and extent of mitotic activity are helpful in the differential diagnosis.

2.2.4 Dermatofibrosarcoma Protuberans

2.2.5 Malignant Fibrous Histiocytoma

This tumour is the second most common sarcoma of the vulva, usually presenting as a large mass in a middle-aged woman.

2.2.6 Epithelioid Sarcoma

A sarcoma characterized by the presence of nodules composed of large cells resembling squamous cells and epithelioid cells; often the nodules are centrally necrotic.

2.2.7 Malignant Rhabdoid Tumour

A sarcoma of uncertain origin with variable microscopic features, the most distinctive of which is the presence of large, polygonal tumour cells with eccentric nuclei and eosinophilic cytoplasmic inclusions; the inclusions correspond ultrastructurally to bundles of intermediate filaments.

2.2.8 Malignant Nerve Sheath Tumours

2.2.9 Angiosarcoma

2.2.10 Kaposi Sarcoma

2.2.11 Haemangiopericytoma

2.2.12 Liposarcoma

2.2.13 Alveolar Soft-Part Sarcoma

A sarcoma characterized by solid and alveolar groups of large epithelial-like cells with granular, eosinophilic cytoplasm; most of the tumours contain intracytoplasmic PAS-positive, diastase-resistant, rod-shaped crystals.

3 Miscellaneous Tumours

3.1 Melanocytic Tumours

3.1.1 Congenital Melanocytic Naevus

A benign tumour of melanocytes that is present at birth.
    This tumour may be small or involve a large area.

3.1.2 Acquired Melanocytic Naevus

A naevus that appears in childhood and continues to grow with increasing age.
    This lesion may be junctional, i. e., at the epidermal-dermal junction, intradermal, or compound (junctional and intradermal).

3.1.3 Blue Naevus

An intradermal naevus composed of spindle-shaped or dendritic melanocytes that are typically heavily pigmented.
    A subtype is the cellular blue naevus, which has a low potential for metastasis.

3.1.4 Dysplastic Melanocytic Naevus (Fig. 192)

A naevus that exhibits slight to moderate nuclear atypicality, which may be present only in its superficial portion.

3.1.5 Malignant Melanoma (Figs. 193–195)

A malignant tumour of melanocytes
   Malignant melanomas account for 2 %–5 % of vulvar cancers. They usually present as masses, which may be pigmented, in the labia majora, labia minora, or clitoris. There are three histological types: acral lentiginous, superficial spreading, and nodular. Vertical growth of a superficial spreading melanoma can be distinguished from nodular melanoma by the finding of radial growth involving four or more rete ridges adjacent to the former tumour. Melanomas may be composed of epithelioid, spindle, or mixed cell types.
   The thickness and depth of invasion of malignant melanomas should be measured for staging.

3.2 Lymphoma and Leukemia

3.3 Yolk Sac Tumour (Endodermal Sinus Tumour)

3.4 Merkel Cell Tumour

A malignant tumour composed of small, neuroendocrine type cells of the lower epidermis; the cells have scanty cytoplasm and nuclei with finely stippled chromatin.
   Electron microscopic examination demonstrates dense core granules, and immunohistochemical markers of neuroendocrine differentiation are frequently positive.

4 Secondary Tumours

The primary site of a secondary tumour of the vulva is most commonly the cervix, followed by the endometrium and ovary. Occasionally, breast carcinoma, renal cell carcinoma, gastric carcinoma, lung carcinoma, and, rarely, gestational choriocarcinoma, malignant melanoma, and neuroblastoma spread to the vulva. Vaginal, urethral, urinary bladder, anal, and rectal carcinomas may extend directly into the vulva.

5 Tumour-like Lesions and Nonneoplastic Disorders

5.1 Pseudoepitheliomatous Hyperplasia (Fig. 188)

This lesion has been observed in a high percentage of cases of granular cell tumour of the vulva and in a wide variety of nonneoplastic cutaneous diseases. Microscopic examination reveals an infiltration of the dermis by proliferating squamous epithelium, which is characterized by bland nuclei and abundant cytoplasm; careful examination of the tissue adjacent to the proliferating squamous epithelium typically discloses the lesion that has caused the hyperplasia.

5.2 Endometriosis (see Cervix, Fig. 142)

The presence of glands and stroma resembling endometrial glands and stroma in an extrauterine site; histiocytes laden with hemosiderin, hemofuscin, or both may be prominent features of the stromal component.
Vulvar endometriosis is commonly encountered in episiotomy sites.

5.3 Ectopic Decidua (see Cervix, Fig. 143)

Enlargement of stromal cells with the acquisition of abundant cytoplasm, resembling decidual cells of the endometrium.
Ectopic decidua is most commonly associated with pregnancy.

5.4 Langerhans Cell Histiocytosis (Eosinophilic Granuloma; Histiocytosis X) (Fig. 196)

A localized proliferation of Langerhans histiocytes accompanied by variable numbers of eosinophils.
This lesion can present as a pigmented papule or as nodules, which may be ulcerated. The patient may have similar lesions elsewhere.

5.5 Benign Xanthogranuloma

A self-limited lesion composed predominantly of histocytes containing minimal to large amounts of lipid.

This lesion appears as multiple yellow to yellow-brown papules, plaques, or nodules, most commonly in newborns. Sites other than the vulva may also be involved.

5.6 Verruciform Xanthoma

A benign warty lesion characterized by an accumulation of lipid-laden histiocytes in the papillary dermis.

This lesion occurs rarely in the vulva in women of reproductive age as single or multiple lesions ranging in diameter from 2 to over 10 mm.

5.7 Desmoid Tumour (Fibromatosis)

A benign, locally infiltrating fibromatous proliferation without atypia and with no more than rare mitotic figures.

5.8 Sclerosing Lipogranuloma

A granulomatous reaction to large globules of lipid; the reactive stroma may become dense and hyalinized.

This lesion, which presents as a subcutaneous mass, is usually secondary to the injection of oily material.

5.9 Nodular Fasciitis

A benign subcutaneous lesion composed of spindle-shaped cells of myofibroblastic type and proliferating capillaries; the lesion may undergo a myxoid change.

5.10 Naevus Lipomatosus Superficialis

A hamartoma composed of mature fat that forms a plaque-like lesion in the superficial dermis.

5.11 Crohn Disease

Ulcerated lesions typically containing noncaseating granulomas occurring in association with Crohn disease of the intestine.

5.12 Cysts

5.12.1 Bartholin Duct Cyst (Fig. 197)

Dilatation of a Bartholin gland duct that is usually lined by mucinous epithelium, but sometimes by metaplastic squamous epithelium.

5.12.2 Mucinous Cyst

A cyst lined by mucinous epithelium, occasionally with focal squamous metaplasia, that is not of Bartholin gland duct origin.

This lesion is typically found in the vestibule and is thought to arise from a minor vestibular gland.

5.12.3 Epidermal Cyst (Fig. 198)

A superficial cyst lined by keratinizing stratified squamous epithelium.

This cyst is usually 2–5 mm in diameter, lies in the labium majus or the lateral portion of the labium minus, and contains cheesy keratinous debris.

5.12.4 Mesonephric Cyst (Wolffian Duct Cyst; Gartner Duct Cyst)

A cyst lined by mesonephric type cuboidal epithelium.

This lesion is typically located in the lateral portion of the vulva, is usually solitary and thin-walled, and contains clear fluid.

5.12.5 Ciliated Cyst

A cyst lined by ciliated columnar cells and occasionally secretory cells similar to those of tubal epithelium.

5.12.6 Mesothelial Cyst (Cyst of the Canal of Nuck)

A cyst lined by mesothelium and located in the superior and lateral portion of a labium majus at the insertion of the round ligament.

This lesion is often associated with an inguinal hernia.

5.12.7 Paraurethral Cyst

A cyst lined by transitional epithelium lateral to the urethral meatus.

5.13 Other Epithelial Disorders

5.13.1 Lichen Sclerosus (Fig. 199)

A dermatosis of unknown cause characterized by progressive thinning of the squamous epithelium, subepithelial edema with fibrin deposition and subsequent fibrosis, and an underlying band of chronic inflammatory cells parallel to the squamous epithelium.

This lesion is the most common dermatosis of the vulva, occurring at all ages but most often in women of reproductive age and older. The lesion may affect the entire anogenital area as well as other cutaneous sites. The vulvar lesions are typically depigmented and plaque-like; in advanced cases the skin has a parchment-like appearance. Ecchymoses as a result of scratching, bullae, and ulcers may be present. Lichen sclerosus may occur in pure form or may be associated with squamous cell hyperplasia, dysplasia, or carcinoma, which, if present, should be diagnosed additionally.

5.13.2 Squamous Cell Hyperplasia (Fig. 200)

Hyperplasia of the squamous epithelium with acanthosis and often hyperkeratosis but without epithelial atypia, significant associated inflammation, or evidence of a specific dermatosis or dermatitis.

Squamous cell hyperplasia usually presents as a discrete white lesion that is plaque-like and seldom extensive; it may be dark red.

5.13.3 Other Forms of Dermatosis and Dermatitis

Many cutaneous disorders affect the vulva, for example, eczematous dermatitis, psoriasis, lichen planus, lichen simplex chronicus, and *Candida* infection.

Unless otherwise stated, all the preparations shown in the photomicrographs reproduced on the following pages were stained with haematoxylin-eosin.

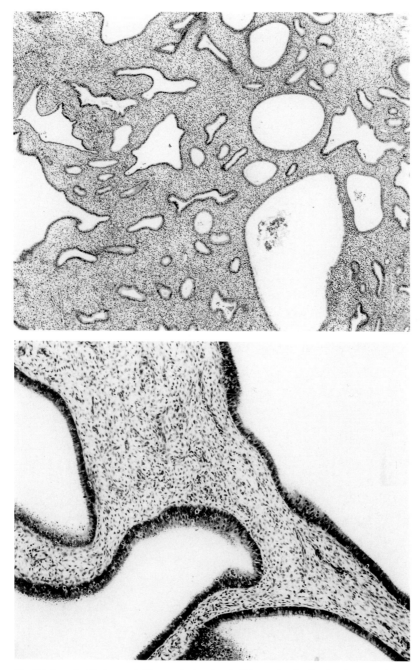

Fig. 1 (above). *Endometrial hyperplasia, simple.* Hyperplastic glands of unequal size, some of which are cystically dilated

Fig. 2 (below). *Endometrial hyperplasia, simple.* Proliferative type epithelium lining cystically dilated glands. Compare proliferative stroma with that of an endometrial polyp (Fig. 8)

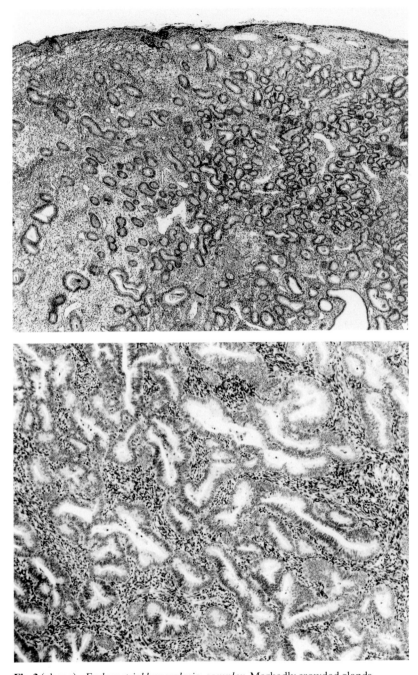

Fig. 3 (above). *Endometrial hyperplasia, complex.* Markedly crowded glands

Fig. 4 (below). *Endometrial hyperplasia, complex.* Crowded, architecturally abnormal glands without cytologic atypia

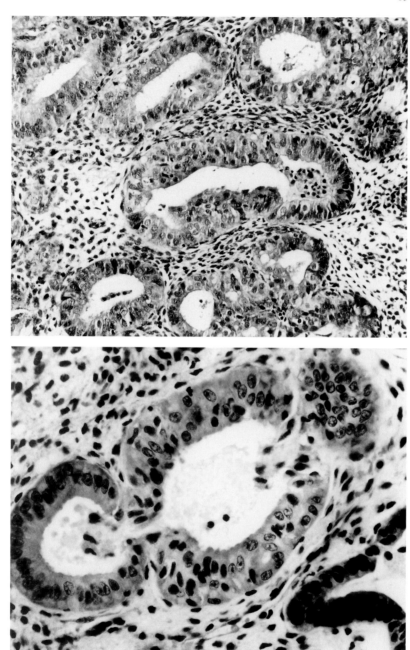

Fig. 5 (above). *Atypical endometrial hyperplasia.* Glandular epithelium showing nuclear atypia and loss of polarity

Fig. 6 (below). *Atypical endometrial hyperplasia.* Atypical gland with large, irregular nuclei showing loss of polarity and containing prominent nucleoli and abundant cytoplasm, which was eosinophilic

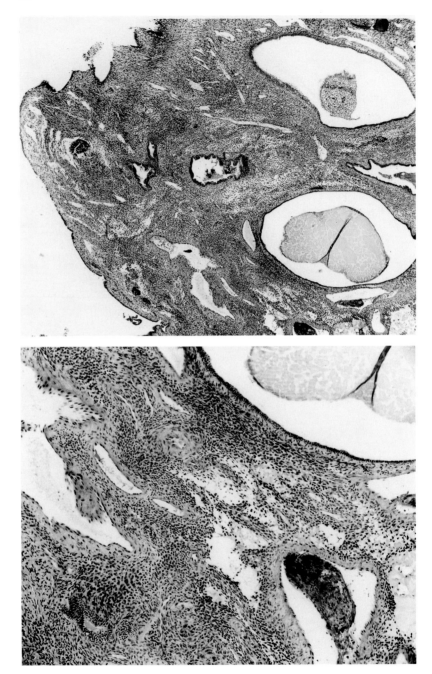

Fig. 7 (above). *Endometrial polyp.* Dilated glands and dense stroma

Fig. 8 (below). *Endometrial polyp.* Higher magnification of portion of Fig. 7, showing thick-walled blood vessels, one of which contains a thrombus, a dilated gland, and dense stroma

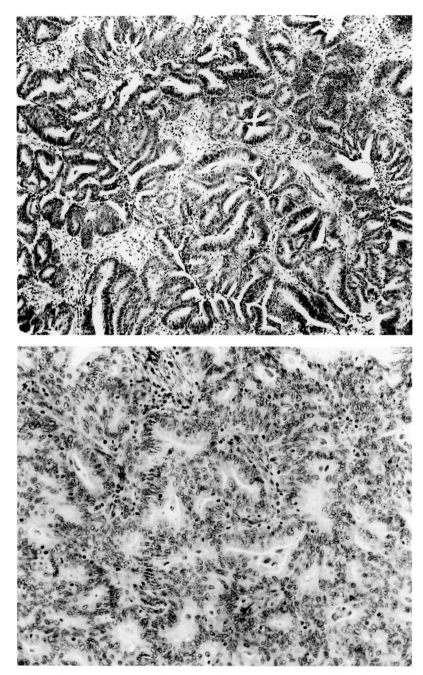

Fig. 9 (above). *Endometrioid adenocarcinoma,* corpus. Crowded endometrioid glands that are back-to-back or separated by fibrotic stroma

Fig. 10 (below). *Endometrioid adenocarcinoma,* corpus. Back-to-back glands lined by cells with atypical nuclei

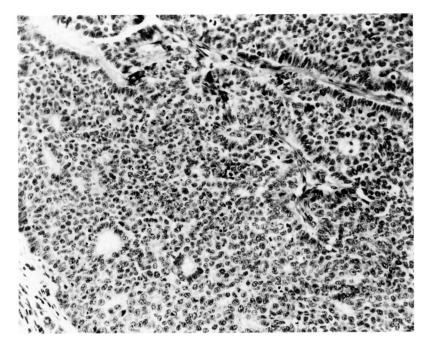

Fig. 11. *Endometrioid adenoarcinoma,* corpus. Solid growth with minor gland formation

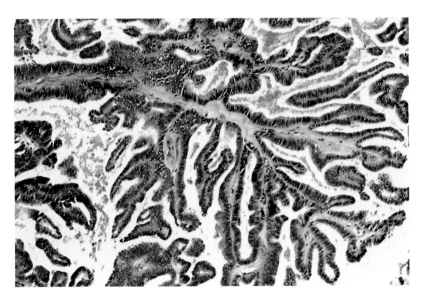

Fig. 12. *Endometrioid adenocarcinoma,* corpus. Villoglandular pattern

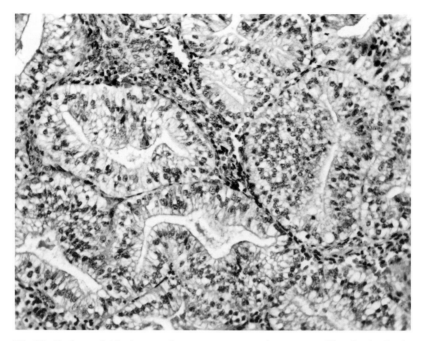

Fig. 13. *Endometrioid adenocarcinoma, secretory variant,* corpus. Neoplastic glands resembling those of early secretory endometrium

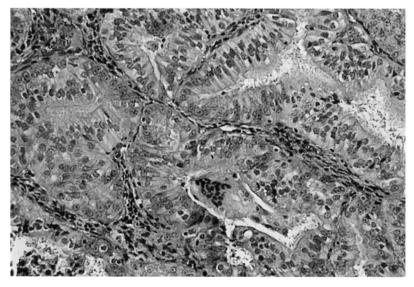

Fig. 14. *Endometrioid adenocarcinoma, ciliated cell variant,* corpus. Well differentiated neoplastic glands lined by ciliated cells

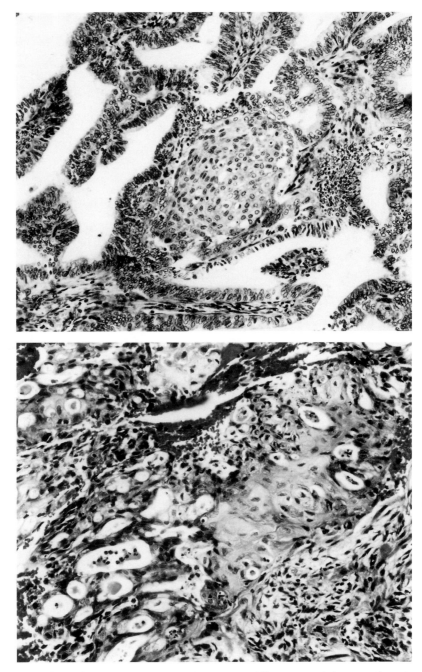

Fig. 15 (above). *Adenocarcinoma with squamous differentiation (adenoacanthoma),* corpus. Intraglandular morule

Fig. 16 (below). *Adenocarcinoma with squamous differentiation (adenosquamous carcinoma),* corpus. Neoplastic glands blending with malignant squamous epithelium, which borders reactive stroma

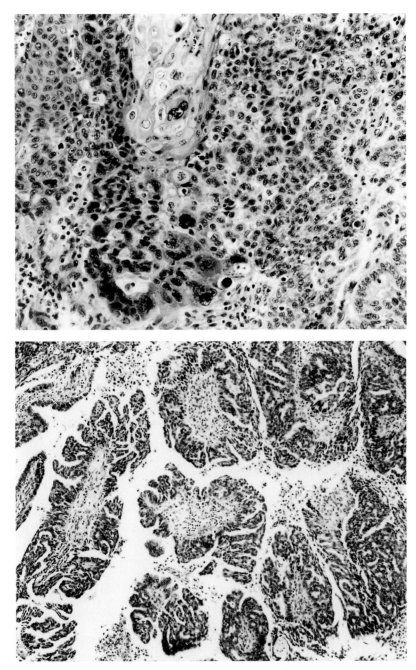

Fig. 17 (above). *Adenocarcinoma with squamous differentiation (adenosquamous carcinoma)*, corpus. Poorly differentiated adenocarcinoma blending with malignant squamous component

Fig. 18 (below). *Serous adenocarcinoma*, corpus. Papillae with fibrous cores lined by poorly differentiated complex epithelium with exfoliation of cells into lumens

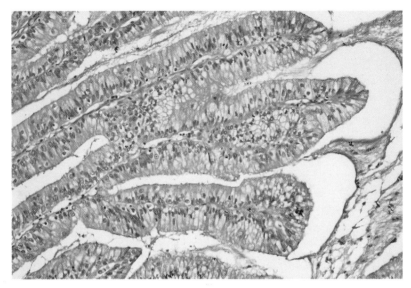

Fig. 19. *Mucinous adenocarcinoma,* corpus. Glands and villi lined by neoplastic cells containing abundant mucin

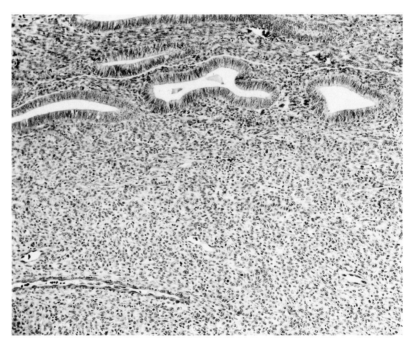

Fig. 20. *Endometrial stromal nodule.* Pushing border between tumour and compressed endometrium *(above)*

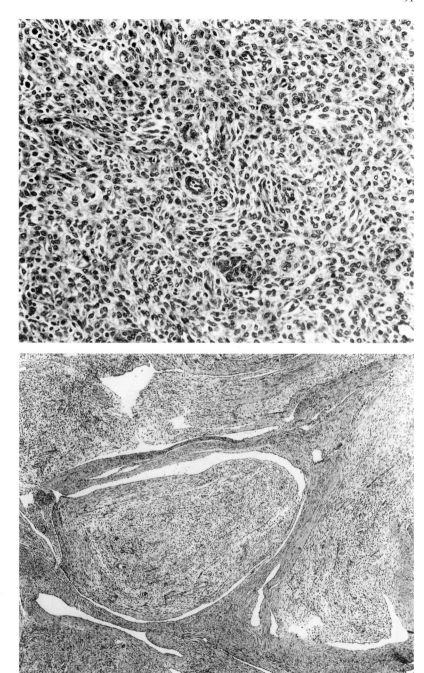

Fig. 21 (above). *Endometrial stromal nodule.* Tumour cells resembling normal prolif-erative endometrial stromal cells whirling around small arteries

Fig. 22 (below). *Endometrial stromal sarcoma, low grade.* Extension of tumour into myometrium and distended thin-walled vessels

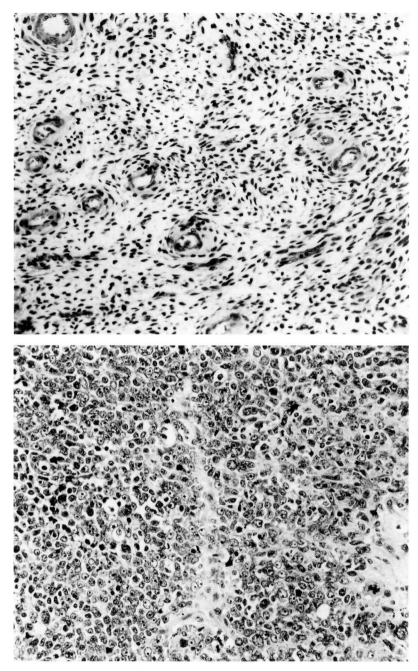

Fig. 23 (above). *Endometrial stromal sarcoma, low grade.* Cells resembling endometrial stromal cells surrounding numerous small arteries that resemble normal spiral arteries

Fig. 24 (below). *Endometrial stromal sarcoma, high grade.* Pleomorphic, mitotically active tumour cells

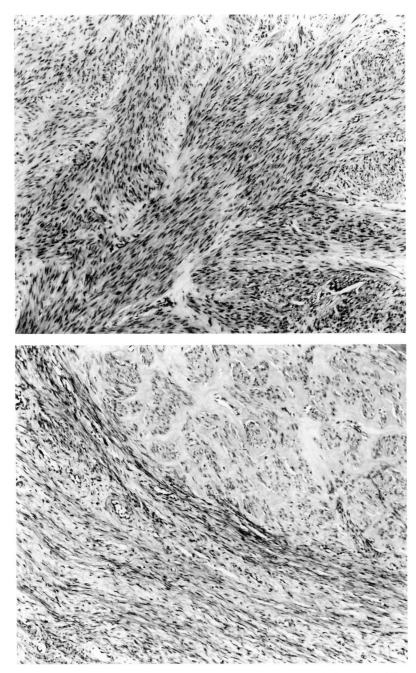

Fig. 25 (above). *Leiomyoma*, corpus. Intersecting fascicles of spindle cells lacking atypia

Fig. 26 (below). *Leiomyoma*, corpus. Hyaline bands separating groups of smooth muscle cells

94

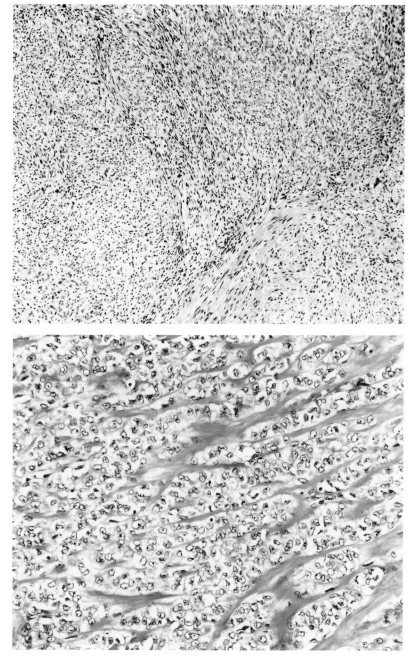

Fig. 27 (above). *Cellular leiomyoma,* corpus. Tumour significantly more cellular than normal myometrium, but without nuclear atypia or mitotic activity

Fig. 28 (below). *Epithelioid leiomyoma,* corpus. Round tumour cells with abundant clear cytoplasm; no mitotic activity

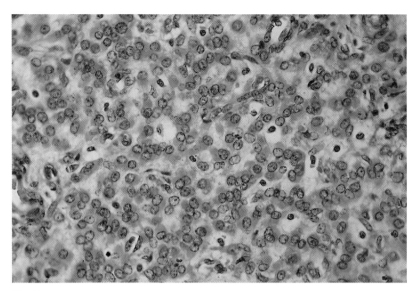

Fig. 29. *Epithelioid leiomyoma,* corpus. Plexiform arrangement of epithelioid smooth muscle cells with dense cytoplasm

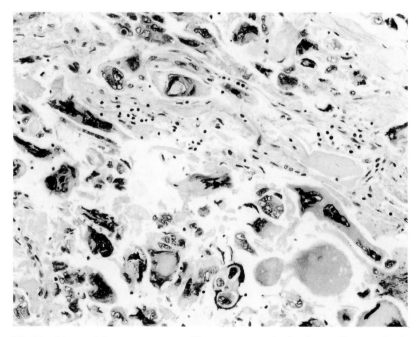

Fig. 30. *Bizarre leiomyoma,* corpus. Numerous symplastic giant cells; no mitotic activity

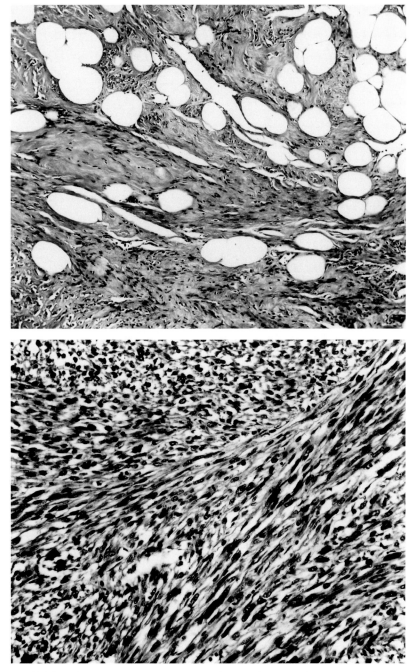

Fig. 31 (above). *Lipoleiomyoma,* corpus. Intimate admixture of smooth muscle cells and lipocytes

Fig. 32 (below). *Leiomyosarcoma,* corpus. Hypercellular tumour with nuclear pleomorphism, hyperchromatism, and mitotic figures

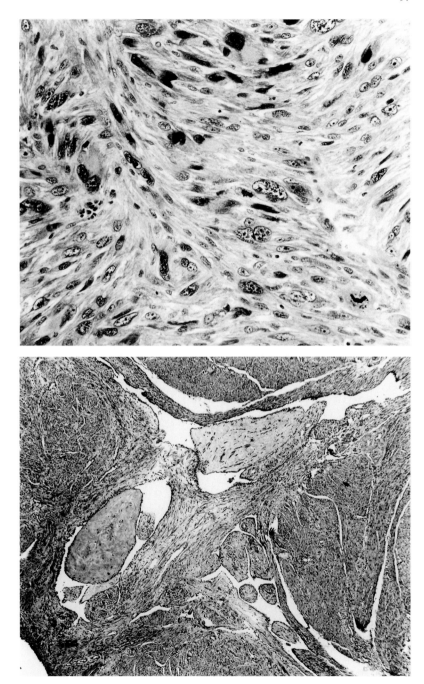

Fig. 33 (above). *Leiomyosarcoma,* corpus. Prominent nuclear pleomorphism and atypical mitotic figure

Fig. 34 (below). *Intravenous leiomyomatosis,* corpus. Cytologically benign, focally hyalinized leiomyomatous tissue within myometrial veins

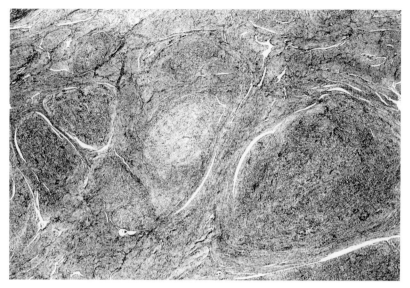

Fig. 35. *Diffuse leiomyomatosis,* corpus. Multiple, closely packed leiomyomas occupying most of myometrium

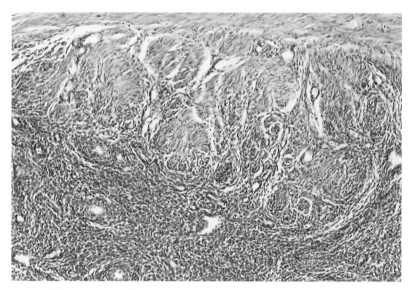

Fig. 36. *Mixed endometrial stromal and smooth muscle tumour,* corpus. Irregularly oval nodule of smooth muscle *(above)* present within otherwise typical endometrial stromal tumour

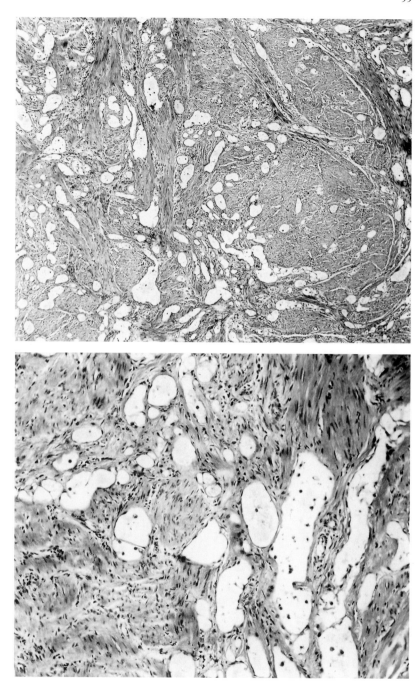

Fig. 37 (above). *Adenomatoid tumour,* corpus. Dilated tubules and small cysts extensively infiltrating the myometrium

Fig. 38 (below). *Adenomatoid tumour,* corpus. Single layer of flattened tumour cells lining tubules and cysts in myometrium

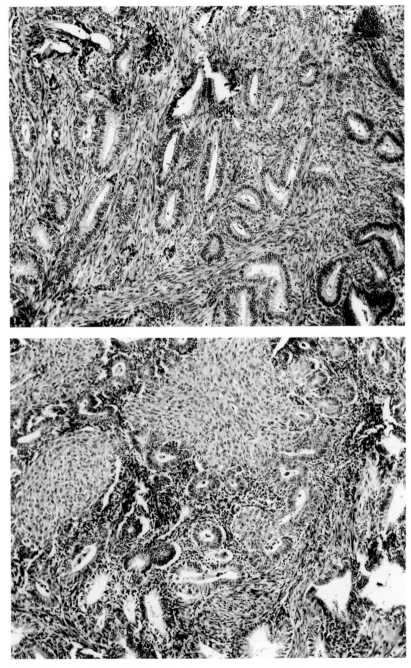

Fig. 39 (above). *Atypical polypoid adenomyoma,* corpus. Endometrial glands separated by fascicles of cellular smooth muscle

Fig. 40 (below). *Atypical polypoid adenomyoma,* corpus. Large foci of morular squamous metaplasia

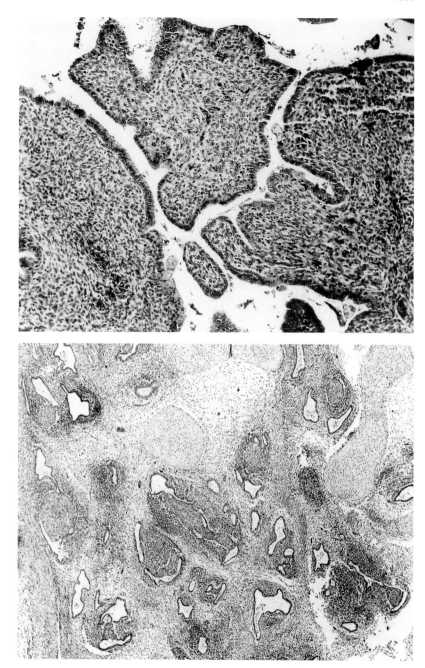

Fig. 41 (above). *Adenosarcoma, homologous,* corpus. Club-shaped polyps lived by benign appearing endometrioid epithelium, with hypercellular stromal component

Fig. 42 (below). *Adenosarcoma, heterologous,* corpus. Glands with focal squamous metaplasia surrounded by dense cuffs of neoplastic stromal cells, and islands of immature cartilage within less cellular stromal component

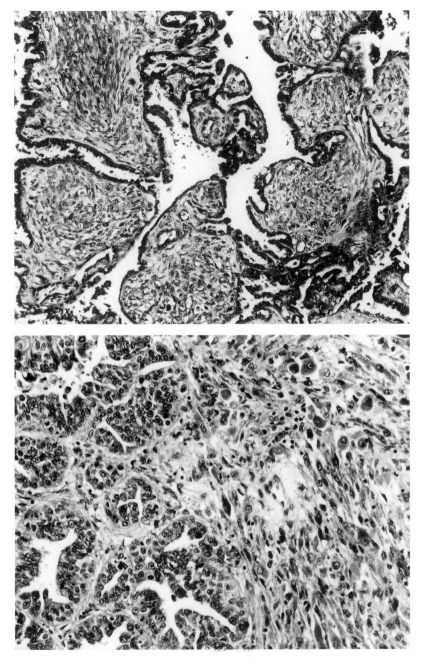

Fig. 43 (above). *Carcinosarcoma, homologous,* corpus. Carcinoma cells with a complex pattern lining polypoid masses of malignant-appearing stroma

Fig. 44 (below). *Carcinosarcoma, heterologous,* corpus. Malignant-appearing glands and stroma containing strap-shaped rhabdomyoblasts

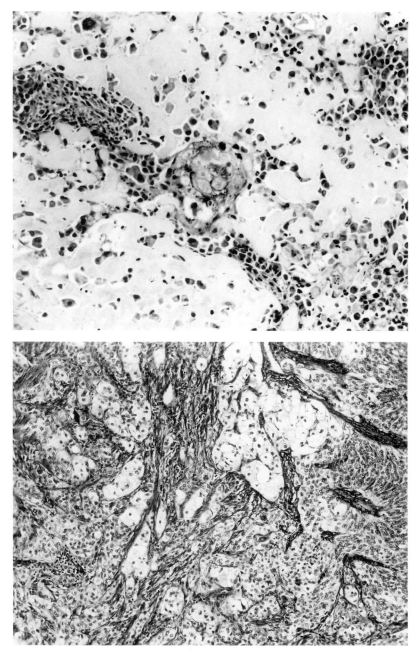

Fig. 45 (above). *Carcinosarcoma, heterologous,* corpus. Large focus of malignant-appearing osteoid and central focus of malignant squamous cells

Fig. 46 (below). *Sex cord-like tumour,* corpus. Closely packed bands of well differentiated cells with an epithelial pattern, some of which have lipid-rich cytoplasm

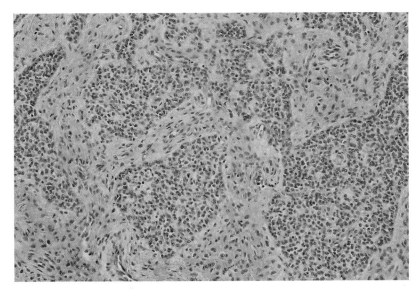

Fig. 47. *Sex cord-like tumour,* corpus. Irregular nests of cells separated by cellular fibrous tissue, resembling a granulosa cell tumour

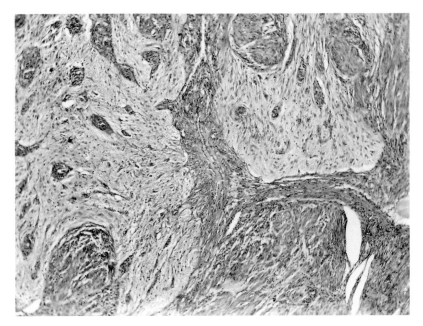

Fig. 48. *Glioma,* corpus. Irregular islands of glial tissue invasive of myometrium

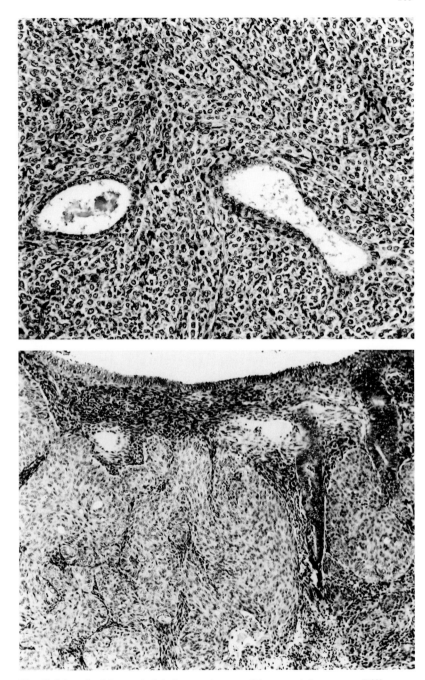

Fig. 49 (above). *Metastatic lobular carcinoma of breast origin,* corpus. Diffuse replacement of endometrial stroma with two residual benign endometrial glands

Fig. 50 (below). *Squamous metaplasia,* endometrium. Confluent squamous morules, which have replaced endometrial glands

106

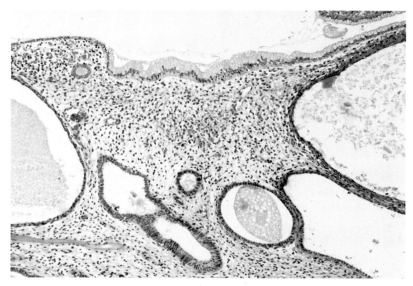

Fig. 51. *Mucinous metaplasia,* endometrium. Surface epithelium mostly replaced by mucin-filled cells

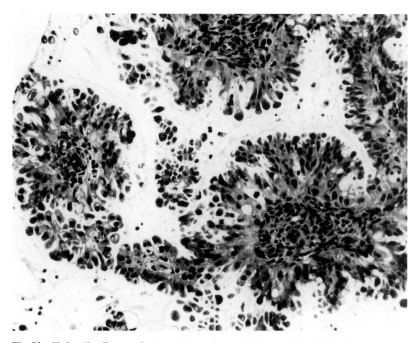

Fig. 52. *Hobnail cell metaplasia,* endometrium. Uniform cells with bulbous, apical, bland appearing nuclei lining adjacent endometrial glands

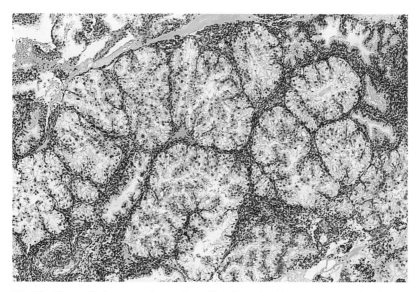

Fig. 53. *Clear cell change,* endometrium. Closely packed hypersecretory glands containing regularly arranged papillae lined by large clear cells (from a pregnant patient)

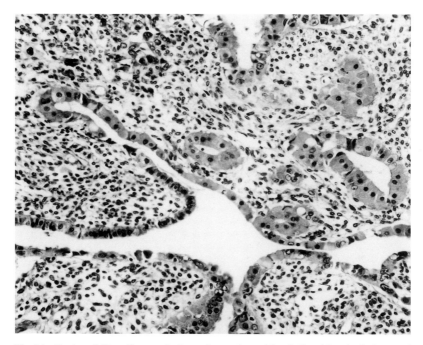

Fig. 54. *Eosinophilic cell metaplasia,* endometrium. Glands lined by single layer of cells with abundant cytoplasm, which was eosinophilic

108

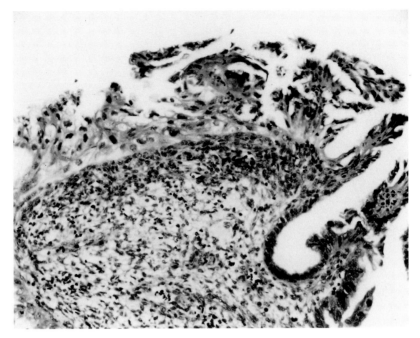

Fig. 55. *Surface syncytial change,* endometrium. Surface lined by an irregularly thick layer of cells with bland nuclei forming microcysts

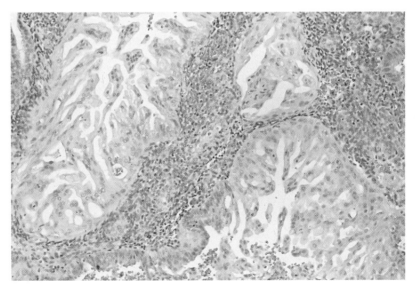

Fig. 56. *Papillary change,* endometrium. Several dilated glands with papillae that are focally confluent and lined by cells with abundant cytoplasm

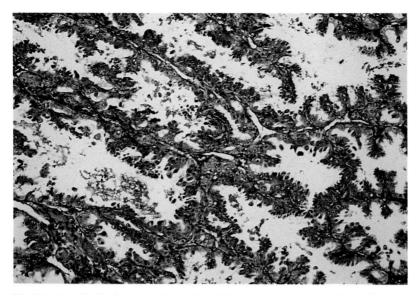

Fig. 57. *Arias-Stella change,* endometrium. Closely packed glands with regularly arranged papillae lined by hobnail type cells

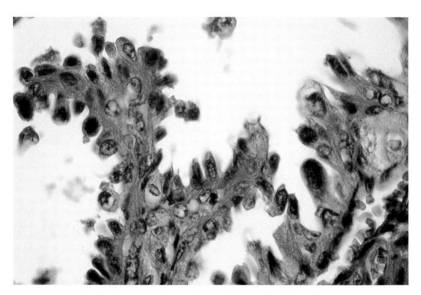

Fig. 58. *Arias-Stella change,* endometrium. Lining cells with bulbous, apical nuclei, many of which have a smudgy appearance

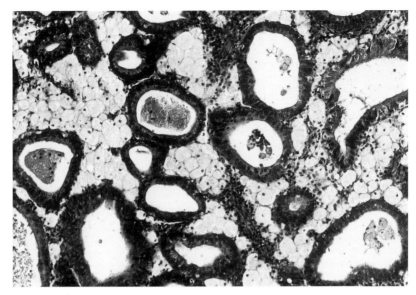

Fig. 59. *Foam cell change,* endometrium. Vacuolated endometrial stromal cells filled with small lipid droplets

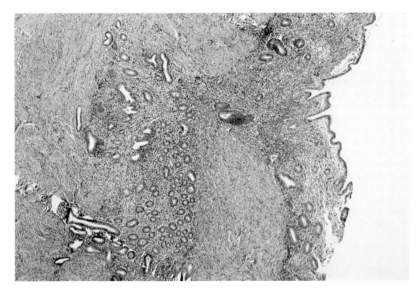

Fig. 60. *Adenomyosis,* corpus. Island of endometrial tissue in myometrium connected to endometrium

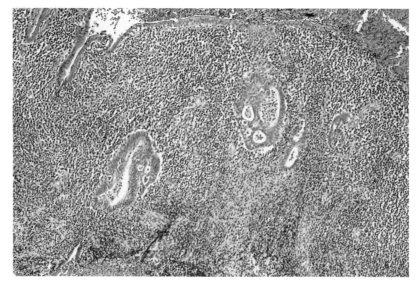

Fig. 61. *Chronic endometritis.* Stroma replaced by round cell infiltrate, which contained plasma cells, and glands that are hyperplastic and architecturally abnormal

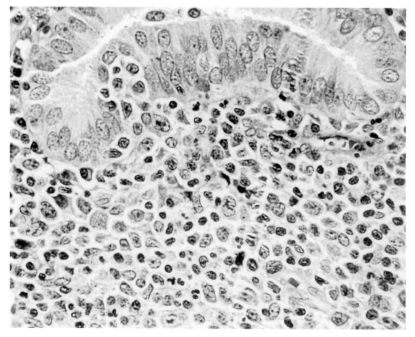

Fig. 62. *Lymphoma-like lesion,* corpus. Polymorphous lymphoid infiltrate occupying stroma and eroding into an endometrial gland

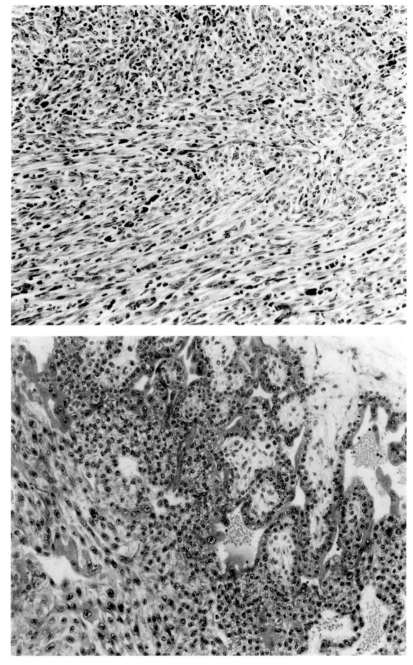

Fig. 63 (above). *Inflammatory pseudotumour,* corpus. Myometrial mass composed predominantly of spindle cells, plasma cells and lymphocytes

Fig. 64 (below). *Sixteen-day conceptus containing of chorionic villi, cytotrophoblast, syncytiotrophoblast and intermediate trophoblast (lower left)*

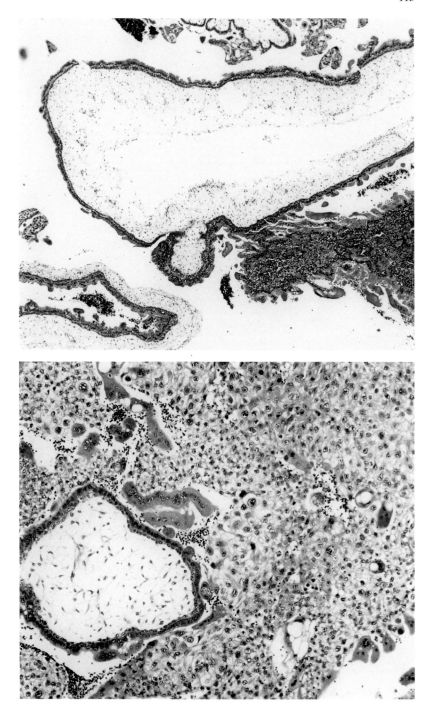

Fig. 65 (above). *Complete hydatidiform mole.* Hydropic swelling with cistern formation and slight hyperplasia of trophoblast

Fig. 66 (below). *Complete hydatidiform mole.* Trophoblastic hyperplasia

114

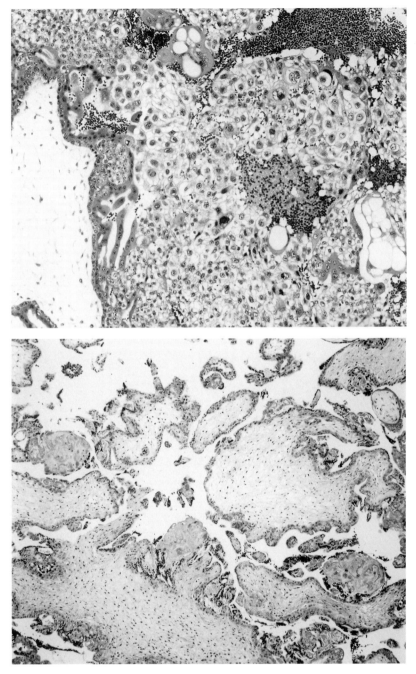

Fig. 67 (above). *Complete hydatidiform mole.* Trophoblastic atypia

Fig. 68 (below). *Partial hydatidiform mole.* Two populations of villi, one normal in size and the other showing hydropic swelling, some with a scalloped outline

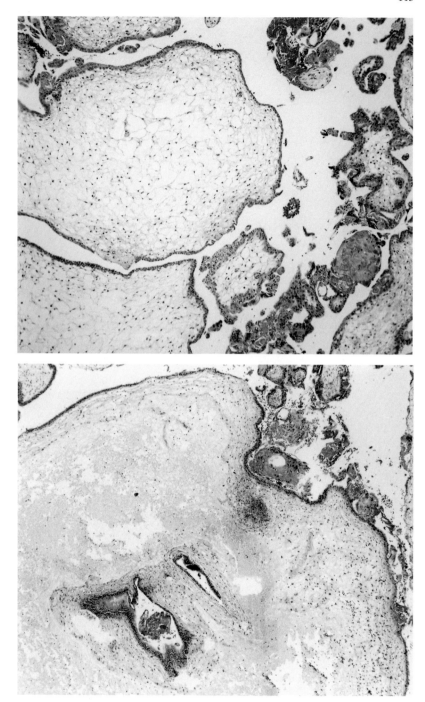

Fig. 69 (above). *Partial hydatidiform mole.* Two populations of villi, one normal and the other hydropic; minimal trophoblastic hyperplasia

Fig. 70 (below). *Partial hydatidiform mole.* Trophoblastic inclusion

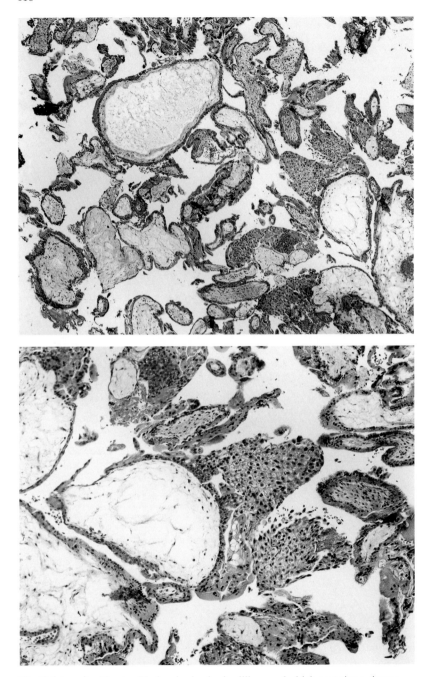

Fig. 71 (above). *Abortus.* Hydropic chorionic villi, one of which contains a cistern

Fig. 72 (below). *Abortus.* Hydropic change and polar orientation of trophoblast, which lacks atypia

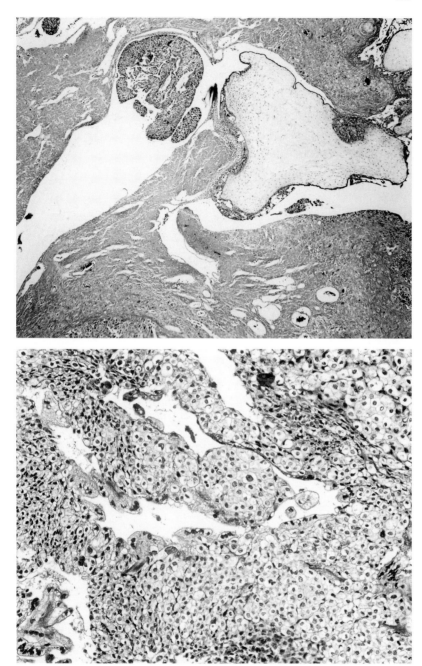

Fig. 73 (above). *Invasive hydatidiform mole.* Molar villus exhibiting trophoblastic hyperplasia and detached nodule of hyperplastic trophoblast *(left)* within vascular space in myometrium

Fig. 74 (below). *Choriocarcinoma,* corpus. Predominant population of cytotrophoblast and intermediate trophoblast; syncytiotrophoblast lining vascular spaces

118

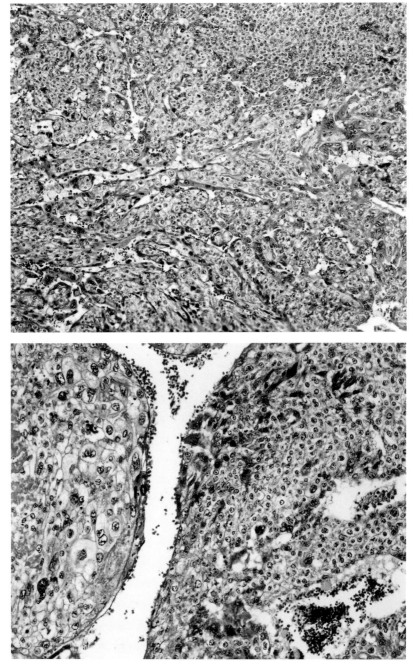

Fig. 75 (above). *Choriocarcinoma,* corpus. Dimorphic pattern of cytotrophoblast and syncytiotrophoblast, with latter lining vascular spaces

Fig. 76 (below). *Choriocarcinoma,* corpus. Cytotrophoblast and syncytiotrophoblast *(right)* and intermediate trophoblast *(left)*

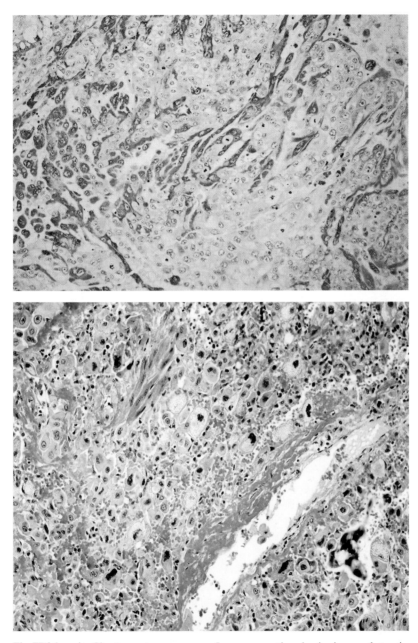

Fig. 77 (above). *Choriocarcinoma,* corpus. Immunoreactive chorionic gonadotropin localized mainly in syncytiotrophoblast and, to a lesser extent, in intermediate trophoblastic cells *(left)*

Fig. 78 (below). *Placental site trophoblastic tumour.* Predominant composition of intermediate trophoblast with single syncytiotrophoblastic cell and fibrinoid in vessel wall *(lower right)*

120

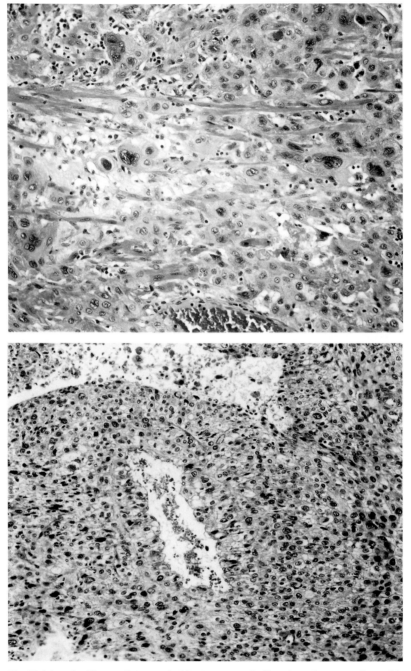

Fig. 79 (above). *Placental site trophoblastic tumour.* Infiltration of myometrium with separation of smooth muscle bundles

Fig. 80 (below). *Placental site trophoblastic tumour (clinically malignant).* Clarity of cytoplasm of some intermediate trophoblastic cells

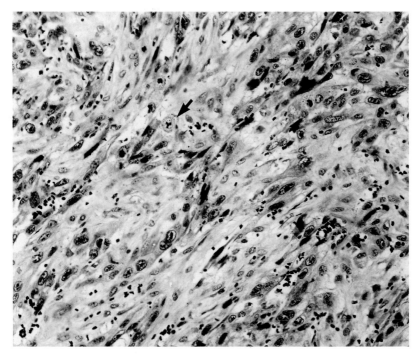

Fig. 81. *Placental site trophoblastic tumour (clinically malignant).* Nuclear atypia and mitotic figure *(arrow)*

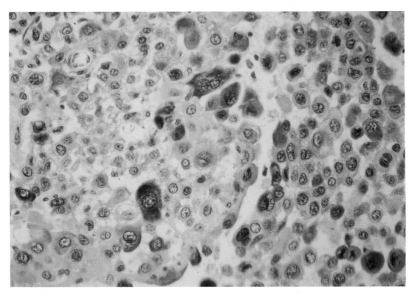

Fig. 82. *Placental site trophoblastic tumour.* Immunoreactive placental lactogen in intermediate trophoblastic cells

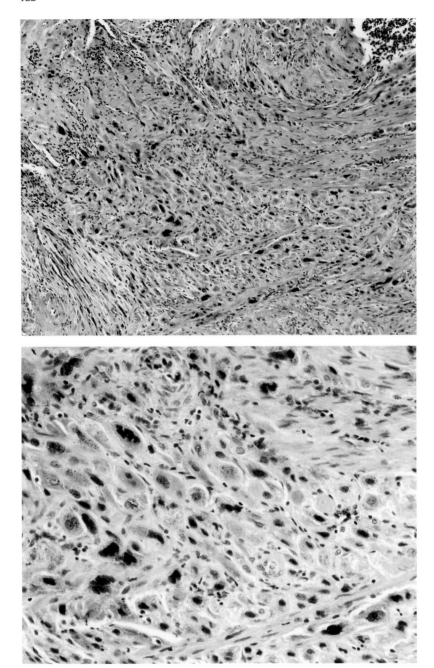

Fig. 83 (above). *Exaggerated placental site.* Intermediate trophoblastic cells without formation of confluent mass

Fig. 84 (below). *Exaggerated placental site.* Smudgy, degenerative appearance of nuclei despite marked pleomorphism

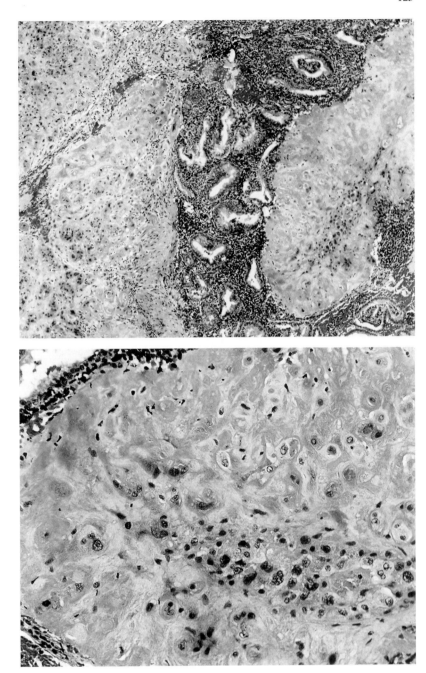

Fig. 85 (above). *Placental site nodule.* Well circumscribed margin and marked hyalinization of two nodules

Fig. 86 (below). *Placental site nodule.* Intermediate trophoblastic cells without significant nuclear atypia

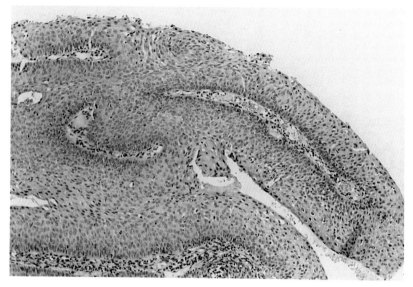

Fig. 87. *Squamous papilloma,* cervix. Papilla lined by thick layer of cellular squamous epithelium lacking nuclear atypia

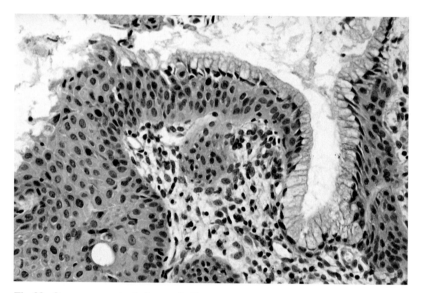

Fig. 88. *Squamous metaplasia,* cervix. Immature squamous epithelium undermining columnar, mucinous epithelium

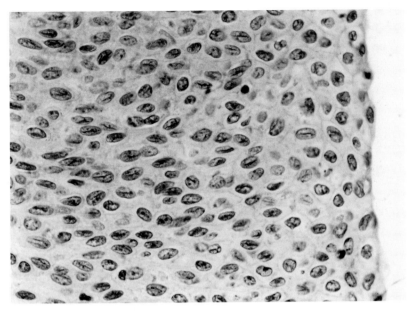

Fig. 89. *Transitional metaplasia,* cervix. Cervical surface epithelium replaced by transitional epithelial cells containing grooved, "coffee bean" nuclei

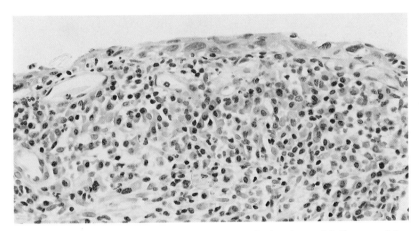

Fig. 90. *Squamous atypia,* cervix. Thin layer of atypical surface epithelium overlying chronically inflamed cervical stroma

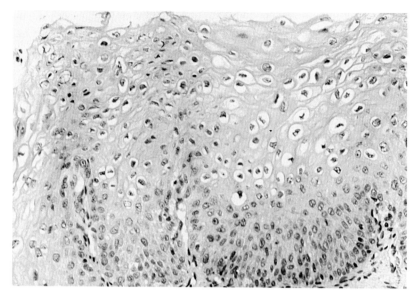

Fig. 91. *Mild dysplasia (CIN1).* Human papilloma-viral changes in upper portion of epithelium characterized by cytoplasmic clarity and abnormal nuclei

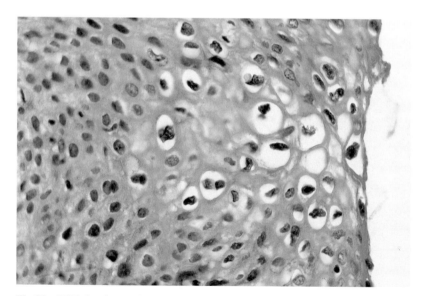

Fig. 92. *Mild dysplasia (CIN1).* Koilocytotic atypia in superficial epithelial layer, characterized by cytoplasmic swelling and clarity, enlarged, hyperchromatic nuclei, and occasional binucleated cells

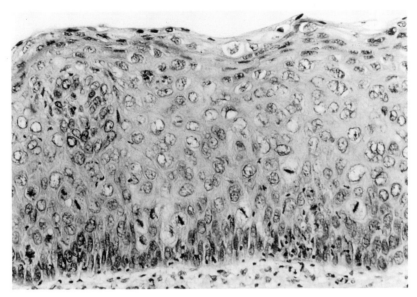

Fig. 93. *Moderate dysplasia (CIN2).* Cytoplasmic maturation and moderate nuclear atypia with numerous mitotic figures confined to lower half of epithelium

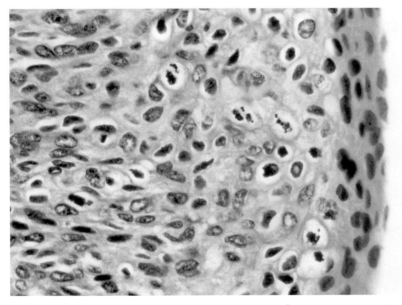

Fig. 94. *Severe dysplasia (CIN3).* Cytoplasmic maturation in upper portion of epithelium and nuclear abnormalities including atypical mitotic figures throughout epithelium

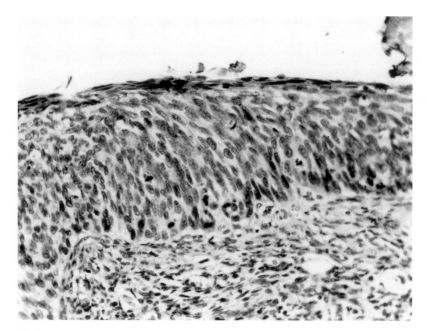

Fig. 95. *Carcinoma in situ (CIN3).* Nuclear abnormalities involving full thickness of the epithelium without cytoplasmic maturation

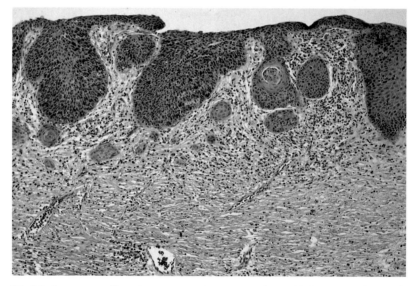

Fig. 96. *Squamous cell carcinoma, microinvasive,* cervix. Multiple buds of differentiating squamous cells extending into superficial cervical stroma

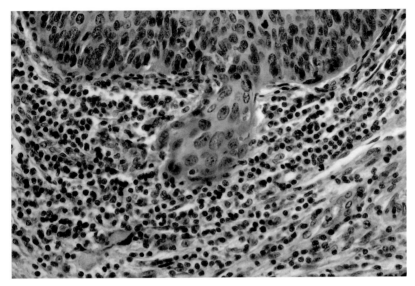

Fig. 97. *Squamous cell carcinoma, microinvasive,* cervix. Single bud of differentiating squamous cells invading cervical stroma from gland involved by carcinoma in situ

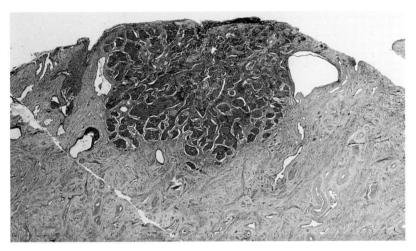

Fig. 98. *Squamous cell carcinoma, microinvasive,* cervix. Measurable tumour mass 3 mm in depth and 5 mm in lateral dimension

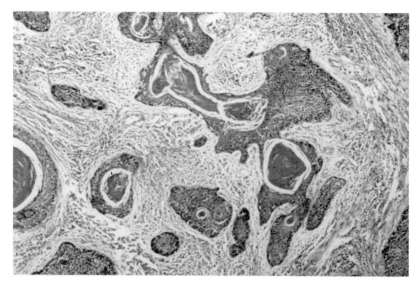

Fig. 99. *Squamous cell carcinoma, keratinizing,* cervix. Irregular, invasive nests of malignant squamous cells, several of which contain central pearls

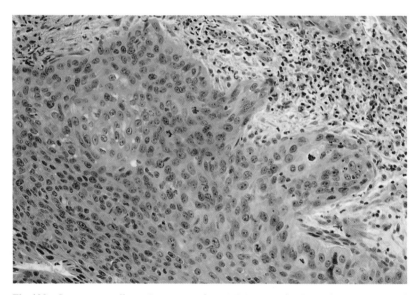

Fig. 100. *Squamous cell carcinoma, nonkeratinizing,* cervix. Irregular aggregate of squamous cells with abundant cytoplasm and without pearl formation

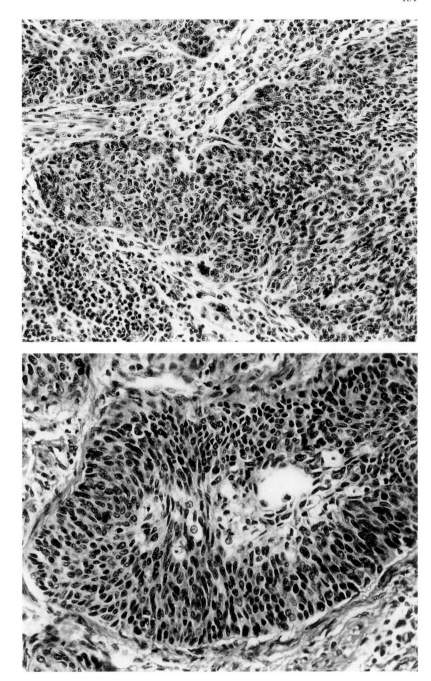

Fig. 101 (above). *Squamous cell carcinoma, non-keratinizing,* cervix. Squamous cells with small, hyperchromatic nuclei and scanty cytoplasm growing in discrete nests separated by stroma

Fig. 102 (below). *Squamous cell carcinoma, non-keratinizing,* cervix. Small squamous cells with differentiation and degeneration in center of nest

132

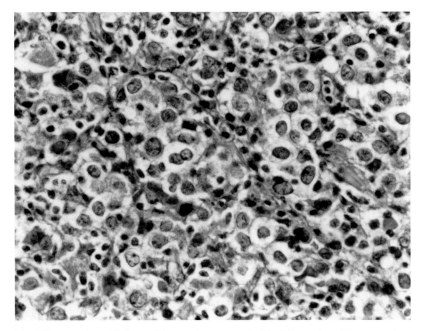

Fig. 103. *Lymphoepithelioma-like carcinoma,* cervix. Undifferentiated large neoplastic cells and extensive sprinkling of lymphocytes throughout tumour

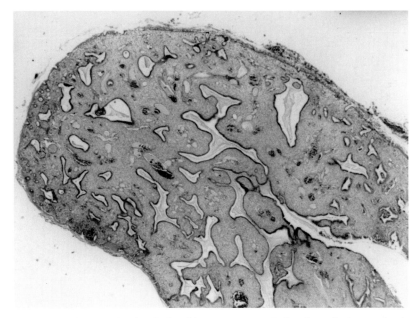

Fig. 104. *Endocervical polyp.* Polypoid mass composed of endocervical-type glands and fibrous stroma

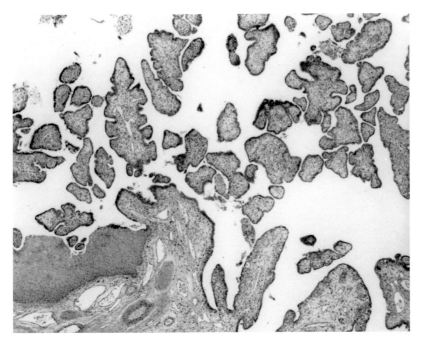

Fig. 105. *Mullerian papilloma,* cervix. Multiple small polypoid projections composed largely of chronically inflamed fibrous stroma and lined by simple epithelium, arising at squamocolumnar junction

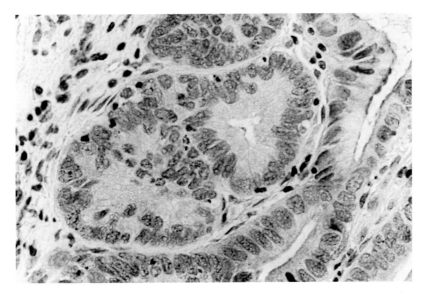

Fig. 106. *Glandular dysplasia,* cervix. Nuclear atypia, focal loss of nuclear polarity and loss of intracytoplasmic mucin

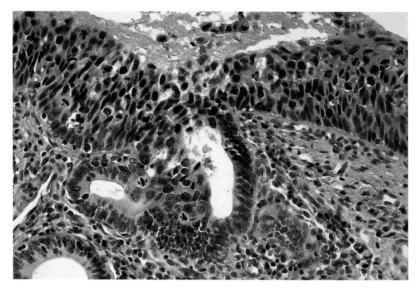

Fig. 107. *Adenocarcinoma in situ,* cervix. Glands lined by highly atypical columnar epithelium merging with squamous carcinoma in situ; atypical mitotic figures

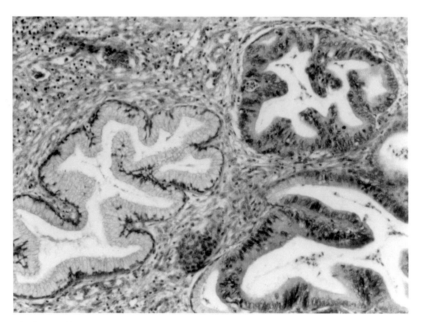

Fig. 108. *Adenocarcinoma in situ,* cervix. Normal endocervical gland *(left)* and glands partly or completely replaced by highly atypical columnar epithelium *(right)*

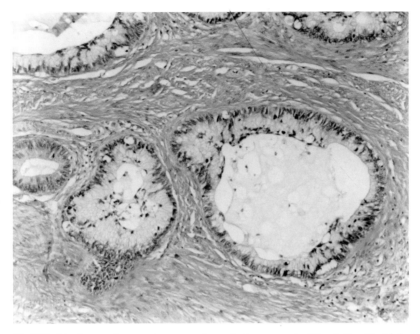

Fig. 109. *Mucinous adenocarcinoma, endocervical type,* cervix. Glands lined by highly atypical endocervical type cells filled with mucin

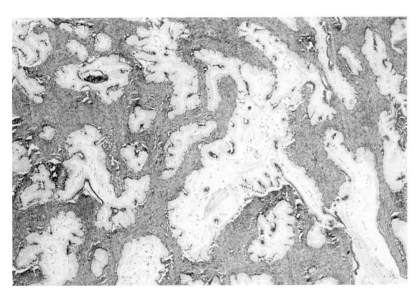

Fig. 110. *Mucinous adenocarcinoma, endocervical type (adenoma malignum),* cervix. Irregularly branching, large glands and small glands lined by mucin-rich cells infiltrating cervical wall

136

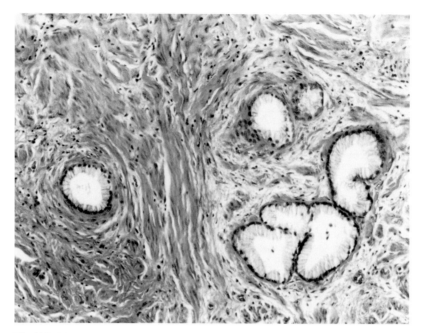

Fig. 111. *Mucinous adenocarcinoma, endocervical type (adenoma malignum),* cervix. Small, highly differentiated glands of endocervical type infiltrating muscle of cervical wall

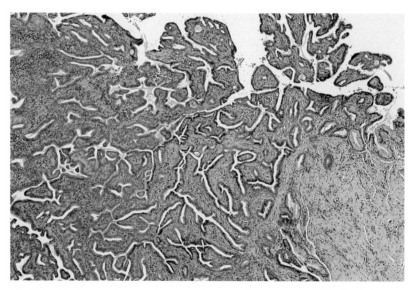

Fig. 112. *Mucinous adenocarcinoma, endocervical type,* cervix. Villoglandular pattern

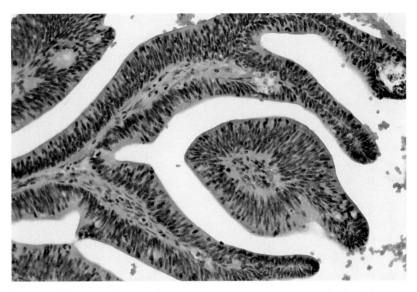

Fig. 113. *Mucinous adenocarcinoma, endocervical type,* cervix. Villoglandular pattern; moderately differentiated, stratified tumour cells devoid of mucin in this area

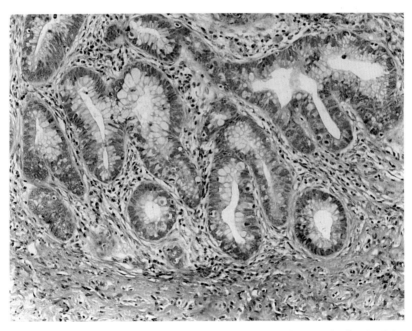

Fig. 114. *Mucinous adenocarcinoma, intestinal type,* cervix. Neoplastic glandular epithelium containing numerous goblet cells

138

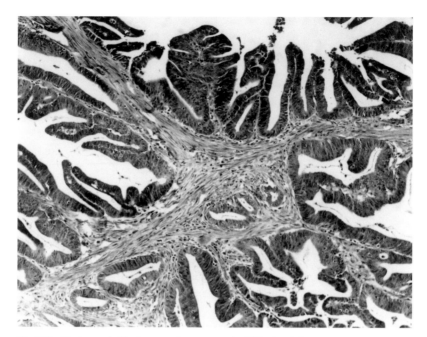

Fig. 115. *Endometrioid adenocarcinoma,* cervix. Villoglandular pattern

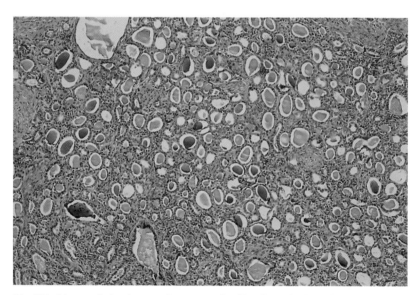

Fig. 116. *Mesonephric adenocarcinoma,* cervix. Closely packed, small, round tubules filled with colloid-like material and arranged back-to-back, resembling normal mesonephric tubules

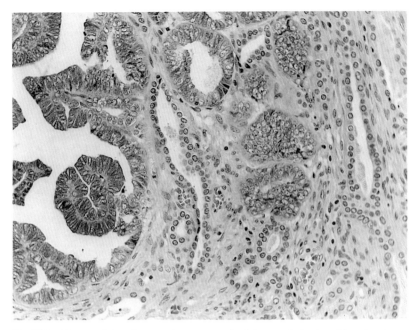

Fig. 117. *Mesonephric adenocarcinoma,* cervix. Mesonephric duct-like structures lined by stratified nonmucin-containing epithelium *(left);* hyperplastic mesonephric tubules *(center and right)*

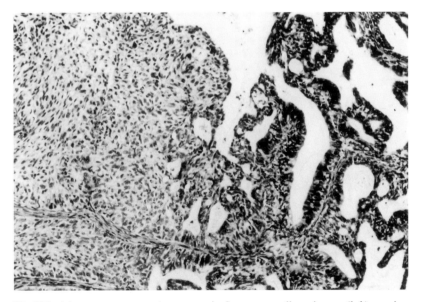

Fig. 118. *Adenosquamous carcinoma,* cervix. Squamous cell carcinoma *(left)* merging with adenocarcinoma *(right)*

140

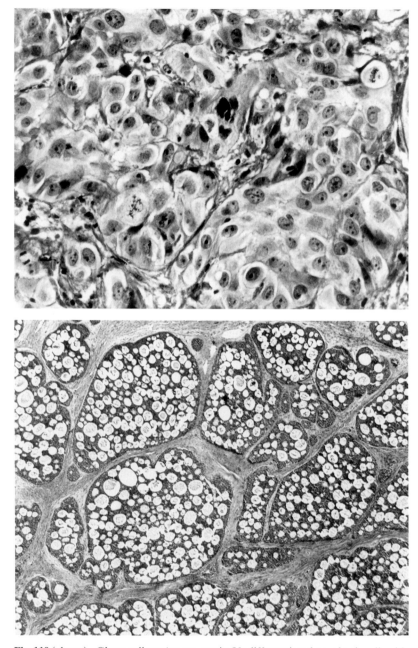

Fig. 119 (above). *Glassy cell carcinoma*, cervix. Undifferentiated neoplastic cells with abundant ground-glass cytoplasm, central nuclei with prominent nucleoli and prominent cell membranes; atypical mitotic figures

Fig. 120 (below). *Adenoid cystic carcinoma*, cervix. Large, rounded nests with a cribriform pattern separated by fibrous stroma

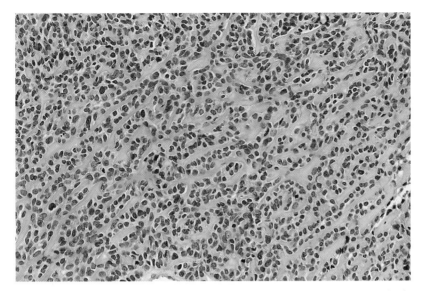

Fig. 121. *Adenoid cystic carcinoma,* cervix. Anastomosing, thin bands of neoplastic epithelial cells separated by cylinders of hyalinized stroma

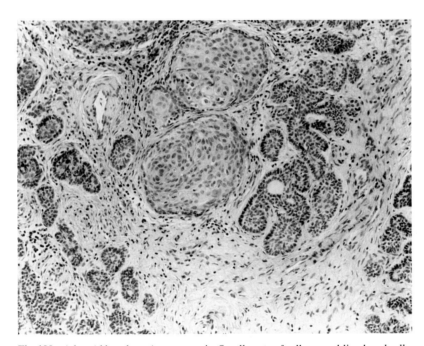

Fig. 122. *Adenoid basal carcinoma,* cervix. Small nests of cells resembling basal cells, containing a few glandular spaces and undergoing squamous differentiation *(upper center)*

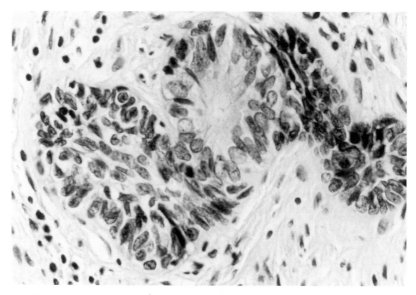

Fig. 123. *Adenoid basal carcinoma,* cervix. Gland formation *(upper center)*

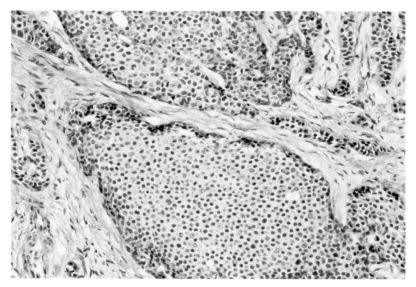

Fig. 124. *Carcinoid tumour,* cervix. Nests and bands composed of uniform cells with round, hyperchromatic nuclei

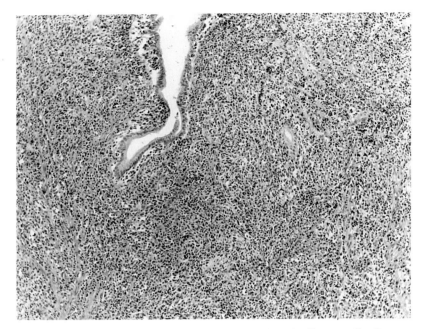

Fig. 125. *Small cell carcinoma,* cervix. Diffuse infiltration of uniform small cells occupying cervical stroma and surrounding an endocervical gland

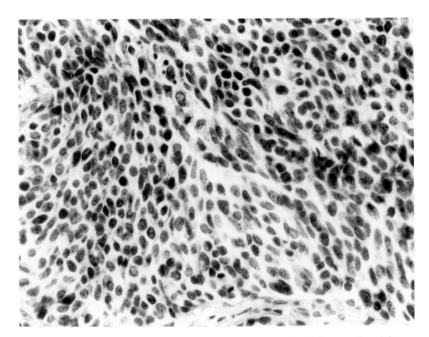

Fig. 126. *Small cell carcinoma,* cervix. Uniform, small, oval, and elongated nuclei containing stippled chromatin and lacking nucleoli; scanty cytoplasm

144

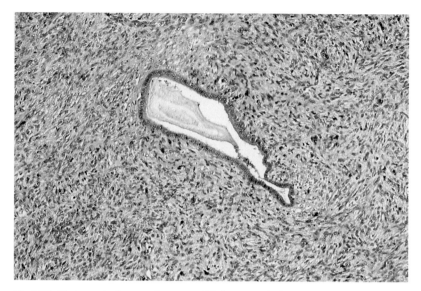

Fig. 127. *Endocervical stromal sarcoma.* Malignant spindle cell tumour without specific features surrounding endocervical gland

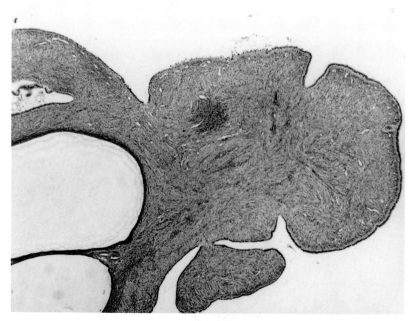

Fig. 128. *Adenofibroma,* cervix. Polypoid growth composed of well differentiated fibrous tissue lined by bland epithelium

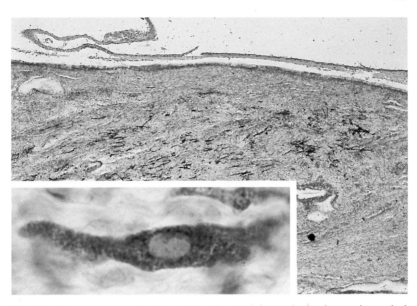

Fig. 129. *Blue naevus, cervix.* Elongated cells containing melanin pigment in cervical stroma

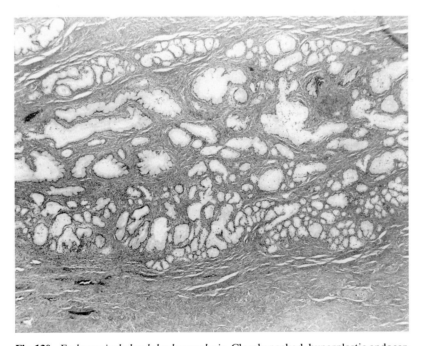

Fig. 130. *Endocervical glandular hyperplasia.* Closely packed, hyperplastic endocervical glands forming a layer sharply demarcated from underlying stroma

146

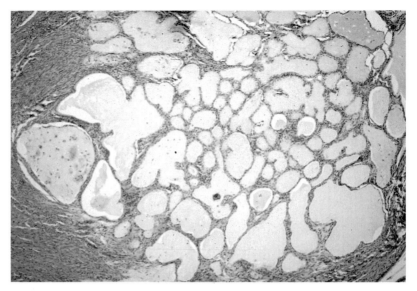

Fig. 131. *Tunnel cluster,* cervix. Rounded aggregate of closely packed, dilated endo-cervical glands

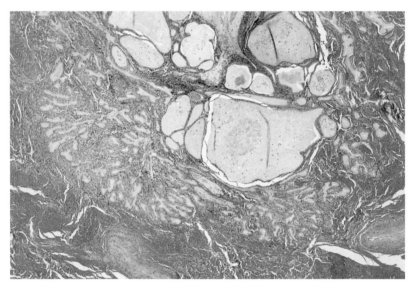

Fig. 132. *Tunnel cluster,* cervix. Sharply circumscribed aggregate of closely packed en-docervical glands, some of which are small and hyperplastic and others of which are cystically dilated

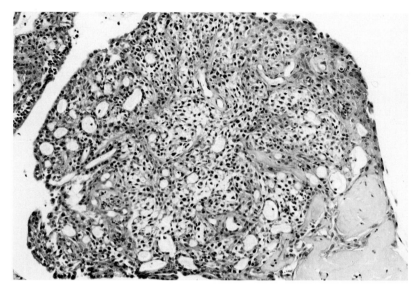

Fig. 133. *Microglandular hyperplasia,* cervix. Polypoid nodule composed of small glands and solid proliferation of loosely arranged epithelial cells

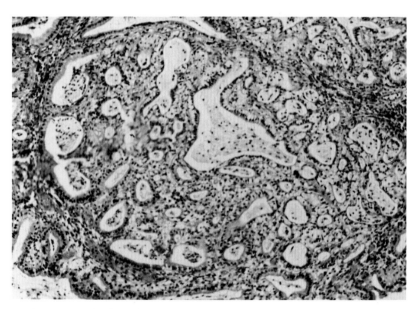

Fig. 134. *Microglandular hyperplasia,* cervix. Nodule composed of mostly small glands containing mucin and acute inflammatory cells

148

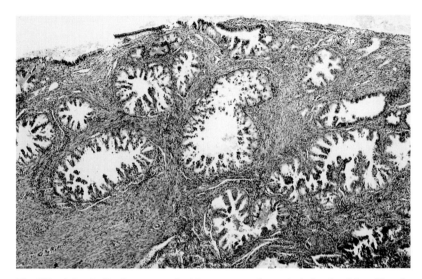

Fig. 135. *Arias-Stella change,* cervix. Numerous endocervical glands with uniformly spaced fine papillae; patient was pregnant

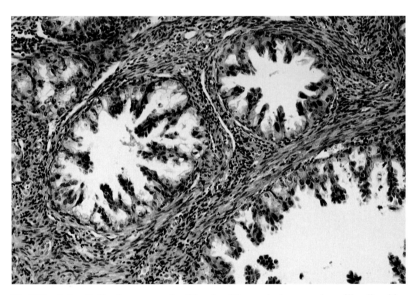

Fig. 136. *Arias-Stella change,* cervix. Glands with regularly spaced papillae lined by hobnail type cells; higher magnification of Fig. 135

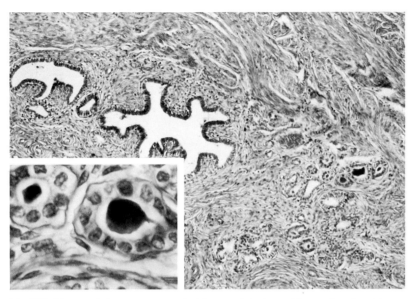

Fig. 137. *Mesonephric remnants,* cervix. Mesonephric duct with pseudopolypoid stromal projections into lumen and mesonephric tubules lined by cuboidal epithelium with colloid-like material in lumen

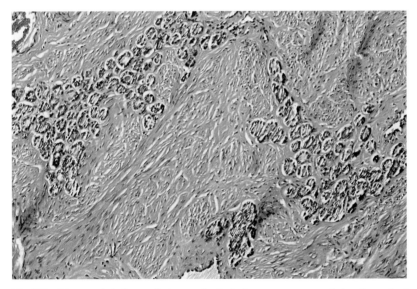

Fig. 138. *Mesonephric hyperplasia,* cervix. Lobular arrangement of closely packed mesonephric tubules in cervical wall

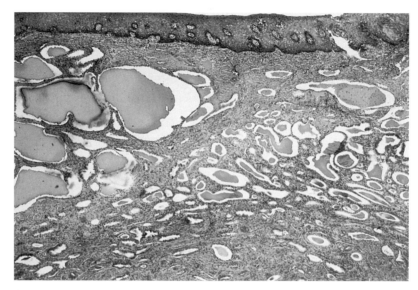

Fig. 139. *Mesonephric hyperplasia,* cervix. Closely packed mesonephric tubules, some of which are cystically dilated, filled with colloid-like material

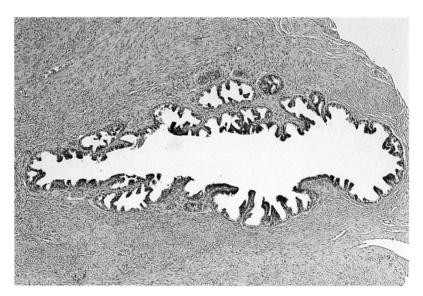

Fig. 140. *Mesonephric hyperplasia,* cervix. Papillary hyperplasia of mesonephric duct

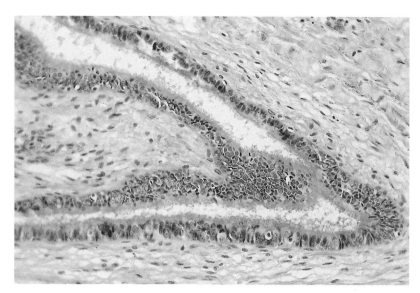

Fig. 141. *Ciliated cell metaplasia,* cervix. Gland lined by pseudostratified, ciliated epithelium

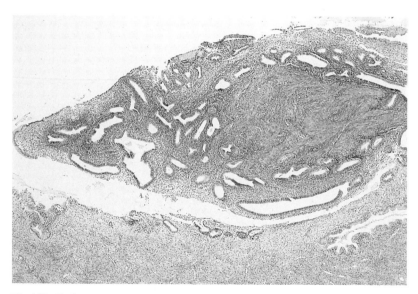

Fig. 142. *Endometriosis,* cervix. Endometrial type glands and stroma attached to endocervical mucosa; large focus of smooth muscle metaplasia of endometriotic stroma

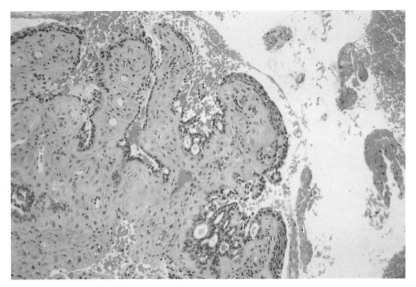

Fig. 143. *Ectopic decidua,* cervix. Polypoid mass composed largely of stromal cells resembling decidual cells of the endometrium

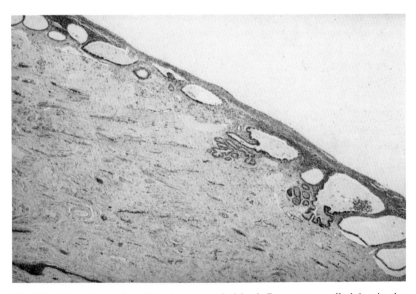

Fig. 144. *Adenosis,* vagina. Glands surrounded by inflammatory cells lying in the superficial lamina propria

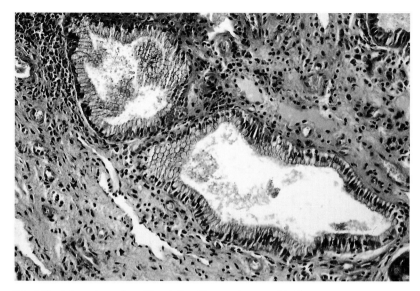

Fig. 145. *Adenosis,* vagina. Glands lined by mucinous epithelium

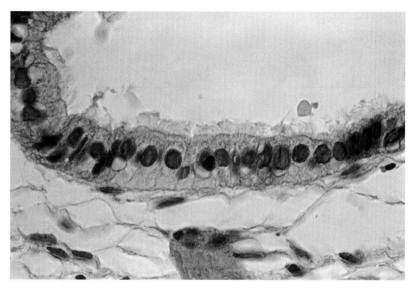

Fig. 146. *Adenosis,* vagina. Tuboendometrial gland lined by ciliated epithelium

154

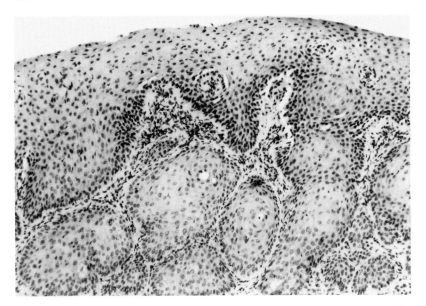

Fig. 147. *Adenosis,* vagina. Glands and surface epithelium completely replaced by metaplastic squamous epithelium

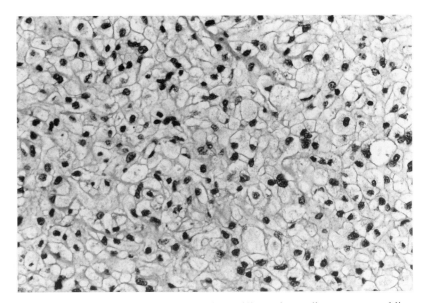

Fig. 148. *Clear cell adenocarcinoma,* vagina. Diffuse, clear cell pattern resembling that of renal cell carcinoma

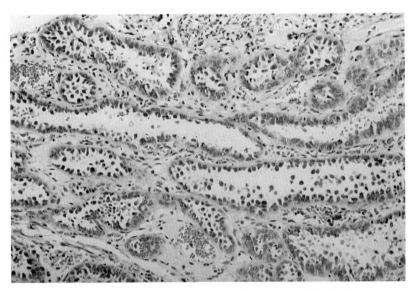

Fig. 149. *Clear cell adenocarcinoma,* vagina. Tubular pattern with tubular structures lined by hobnail cells

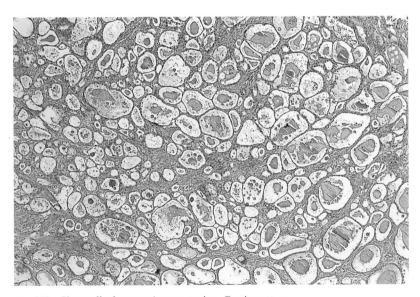

Fig. 150. *Clear cell adenocarcinoma,* vagina. Cystic pattern

156

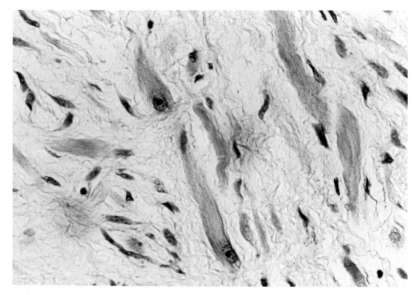

Fig. 151. *Rhabdomyoma*, vagina. Large, mature striated muscle cells in fibrous stroma

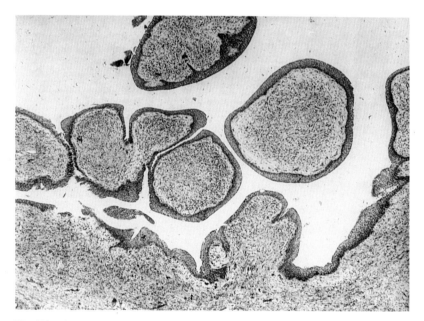

Fig. 152. *Sarcoma botryoides (embryonal rhabdomyosarcoma)*, vagina. Multiple polypoid projections composed of cellular tumour covered by squamous epithelium

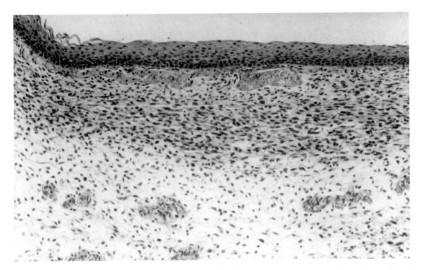

Fig. 153. *Sarcoma botryoides (embryonal rhabdomyosarcoma)*, vagina. Superficial (cambium) layer of cellular tumour and subjacent layer of oedematous tumour

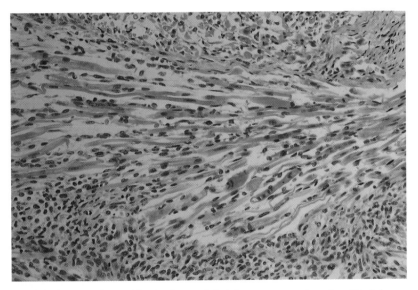

Fig. 154. *Sarcoma botryoides (embryonal rhabdomyosarcoma)*, vagina. Rhabdomyoblasts

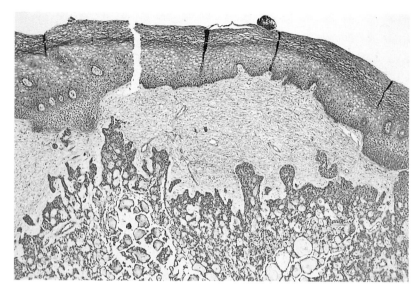

Fig. 155. *Mixed tumour,* vagina. Epithelial component separated by stroma from overlying squamous epithelium

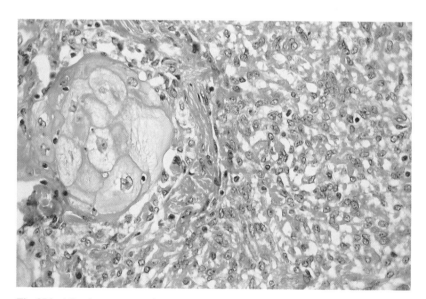

Fig. 156. *Mixed tumour,* vagina. Nest of squamous cells adjacent to predominant small cells of stromal type

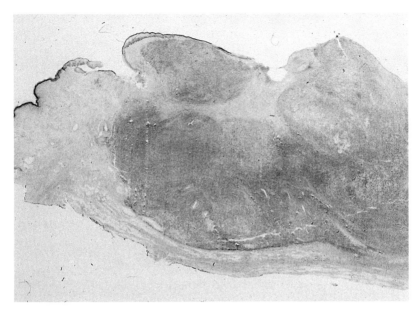

Fig. 157. *Malignant lymphoma,* vagina. Solid mass of lymphoid cells situated mainly deep in vaginal wall

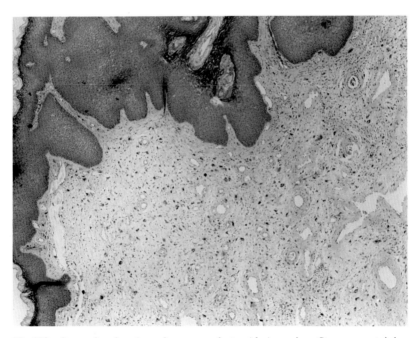

Fig. 158. *Stromal polyp (pseudosarcoma botryoides),* vagina. Stroma containing numerous large cells and dilated, thin-walled vessels

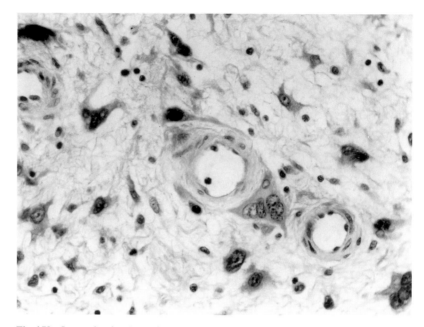

Fig. 159. *Stromal polyp (pseudosarcoma botryoides),* vagina. Star-shaped cells, some of which are multinucleated, with pointed processes; absence of mitotic activity

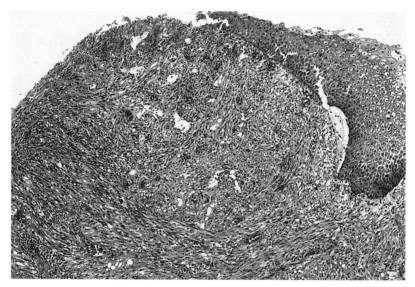

Fig. 160. *Postoperative spindle cell nodule,* vagina. Intersecting fascicles of closely packed spindle cells resembling sarcoma

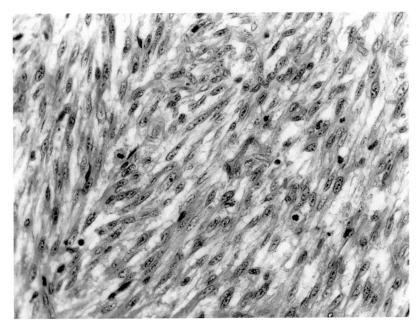

Fig. 161. *Postoperative spindle cell nodule,* vagina. Spindle cells with large nuclei; numerous mitotic figures

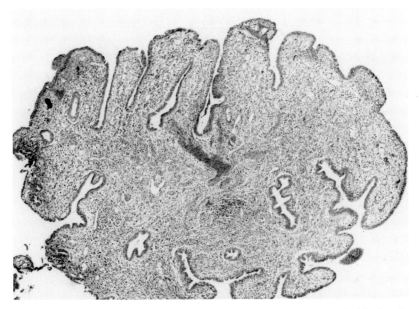

Fig. 162. *Prolapse of fallopian tube,* vagina. Plicae expanded and fused with chronic inflammation and fibrosis of stroma

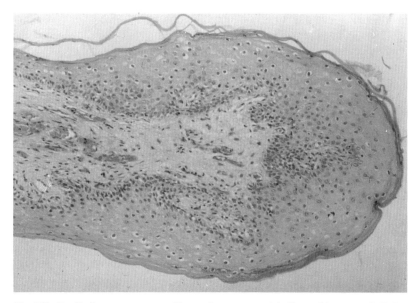

Fig. 163. *Vestibular squamous papilloma.* Squamous epithelium without atypia lining delicate fibrovascular stalk

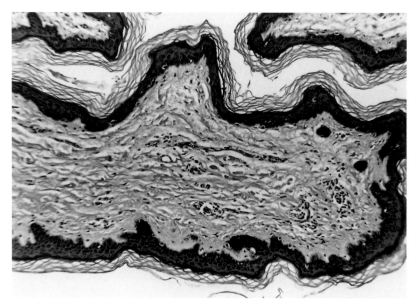

Fig. 164. *Fibroepithelial polyp,* vulva. Polypoid lesion with prominent fibrovascular core covered by hyperkeratotic squamous epithelium that lacks atypia

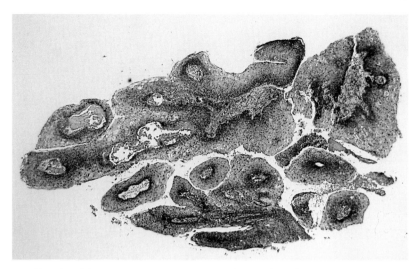

Fig. 165. *Condyloma acuminatum,* vulva. Multipolypoid lesion lined by thick squamous epithelium

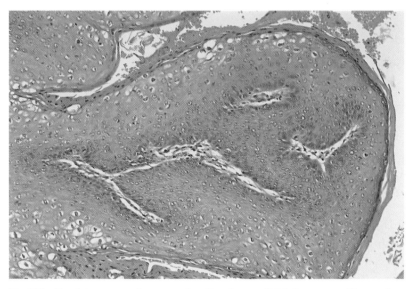

Fig. 166. *Condyloma acuminatum,* vulva. Focal, superficial, human papilloma-virus changes

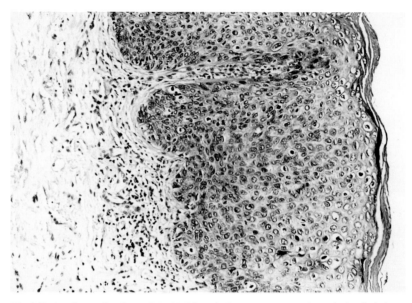

Fig. 167. *Moderate dysplasia (VIN2).* Disorderly arrangement of atypical cells in lower half of epithelium and maturation in upper half

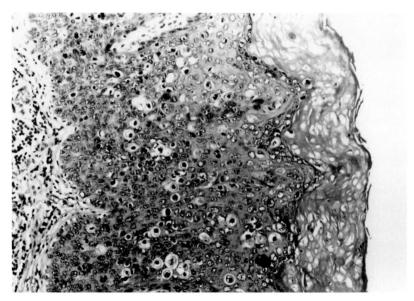

Fig. 168. *Severe dysplasia (VIN3).* Corps ronds with pyknotic nuclei surrounded by haloes; atypical nuclei in upper third of epithelium

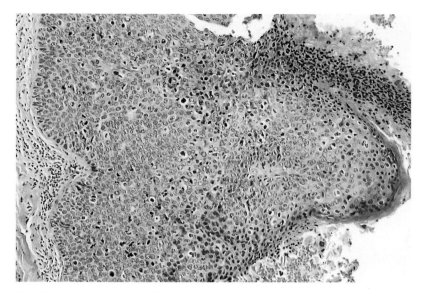

Fig. 169. *Carcinoma in situ (VIN3).* Crowded small cells without maturation occupying full thickness of epithelium

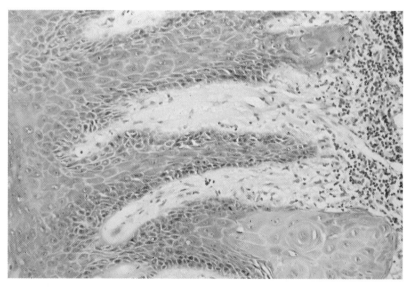

Fig. 170. *Carcinoma in situ (simplex type) (VIN3).* Nuclear abnormalities with abortive pearl formation in papillary downgrowth of squamous epithelium

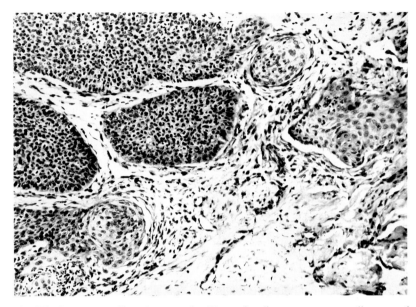

Fig. 171. *Squamous cell carcinoma,* vulva. Nests of malignant squamous cells, some of which are rounded and basaloid and others of which show squamous cell maturation

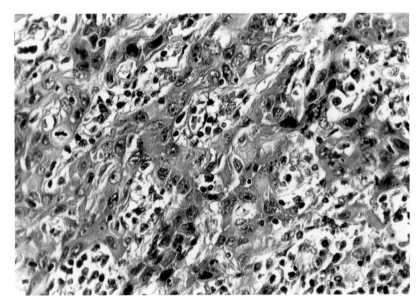

Fig. 172. *Squamous cell carcinoma, nonkeratinizing,* vulva. Anastomosing trabeculae

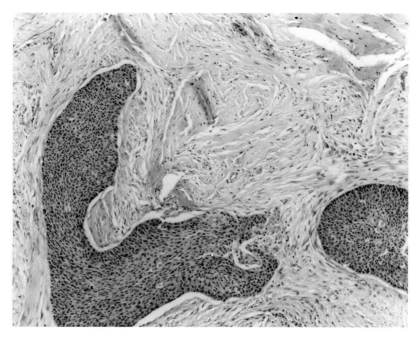

Fig. 173. *Squamous cell carcinoma, basaloid,* vulva. Carcinoma cells resembling those of squamous carcinoma in situ of cervix

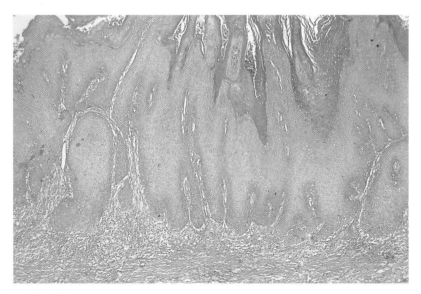

Fig. 174. *Verrucous carcinoma,* vulva. Abundant keratin formation and bulbous downgrowths of well differentiated squamous epithelium

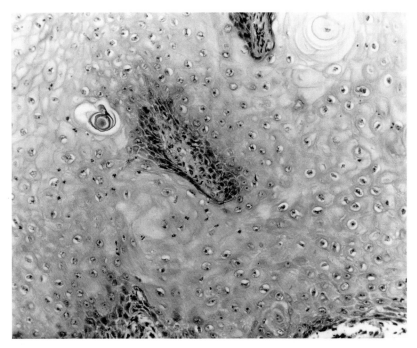

Fig. 175. *Verrucous carcinoma,* vulva. High degree of differentiation of tumour cells

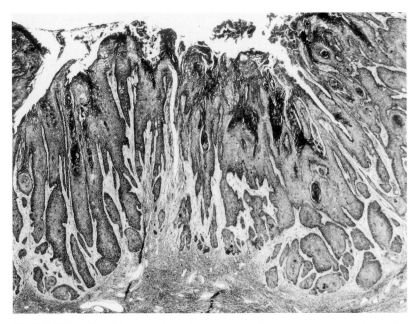

Fig. 176. *Warty (condylomatous) carcinoma,* vulva. Verrucous surface and underlying invasive carcinoma

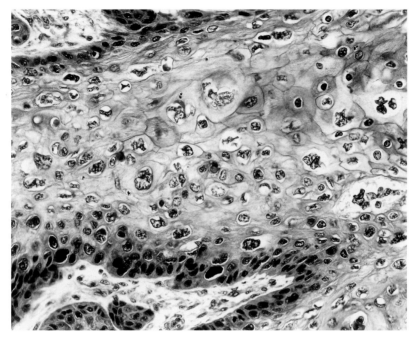

Fig. 177. *Warty (condylomatous) carcinoma,* vulva. Noninvasive component with koilocytosis-like changes

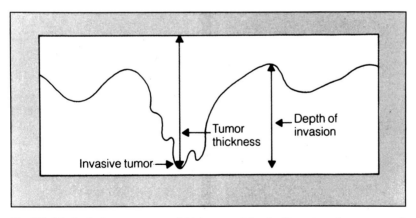

Fig. 178. Method of measurement of thickness and depth of invasion of squamous cell carcinoma of vulva

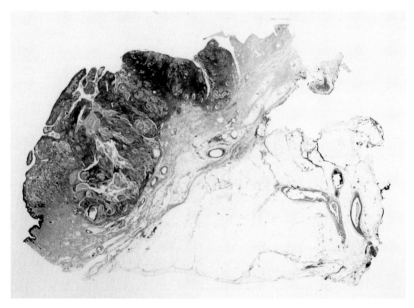

Fig. 179. *Squamous cell carcinoma,* vulva. Tumour 5 mm in maximal vertical thickness

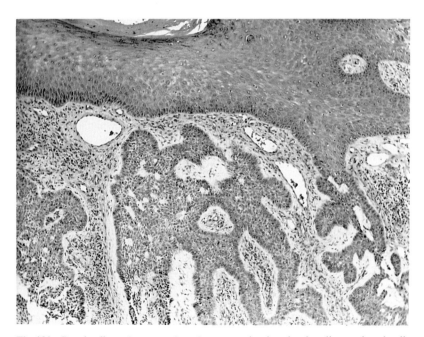

Fig. 180. *Basal cell carcinoma,* vulva. Anastomosing bands of malignant basal cells arising from base of squamous epithelium

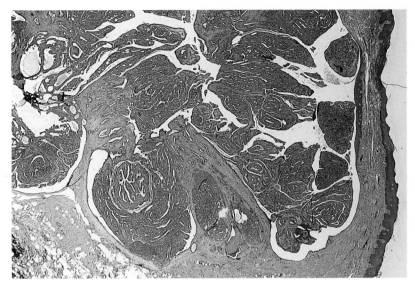

Fig. 181. *Papillary hidradenoma,* vulva. Cystic papillary tumour sharply demarcated from adjacent stroma

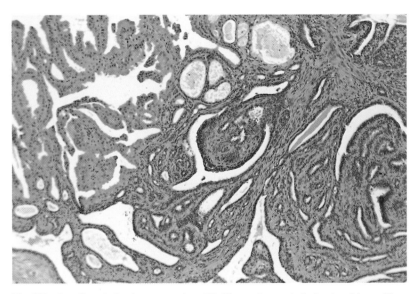

Fig. 182. *Papillary hidradenoma,* vulva. Slit-like and rounded glands with papillae; apocrine metaplasia of tumour cells *(left)*

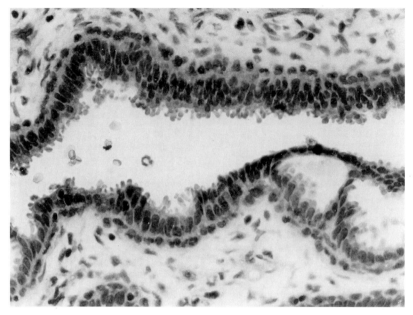

Fig. 183. *Papillary hidradenoma,* vulva. Layer of myoepithelial cells subjacent to secretory cells

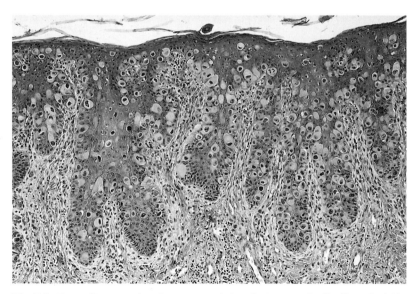

Fig. 184. *Paget disease,* vulva. Large, rounded, pale Paget cells distributed within thickened squamous epithelium

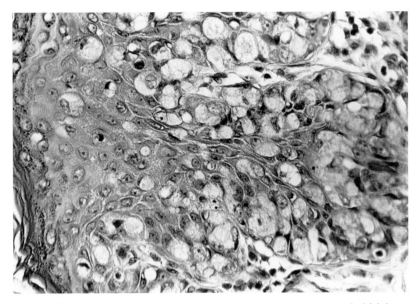

Fig. 185. *Paget disease*, vulva. Paget cells with foamy cytoplasm, some of which have a signet ring appearance

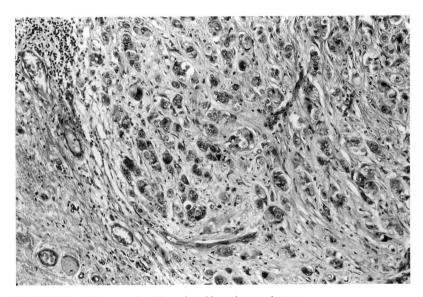

Fig. 186. *Paget disease*, vulva. Associated invasive carcinoma

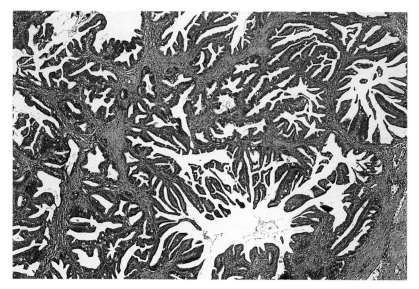

Fig. 187. *Bartholin gland adenocarcinoma.* Papillary pattern

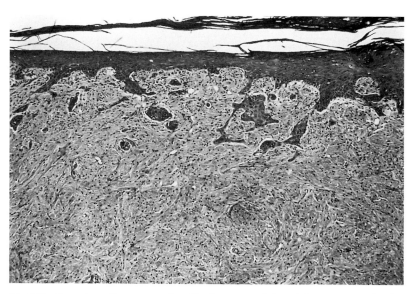

Fig. 188. *Granular cell tumour,* vulva. Replacement of dermis by tumour cells with overlying pseudoepitheliomatous hyperplasia

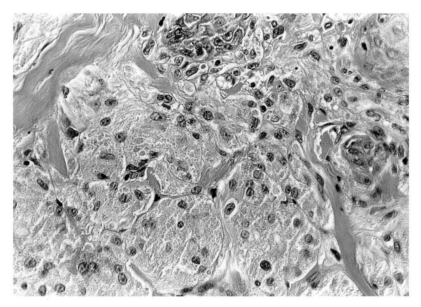

Fig. 189. *Granular cell tumour,* vulva. Coarse granules filling cytoplasm of tumour cells

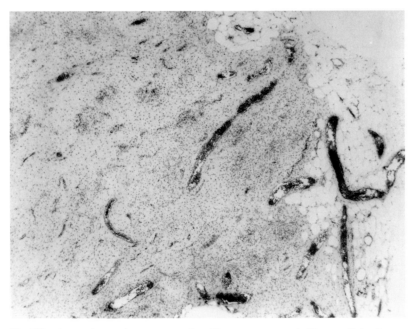

Fig. 190. *Aggressive angiomyxoma,* vulva. Tumour composed of hypocellular, loose, myxoid tissue containing numerous blood vessels and invading fat *(right)*

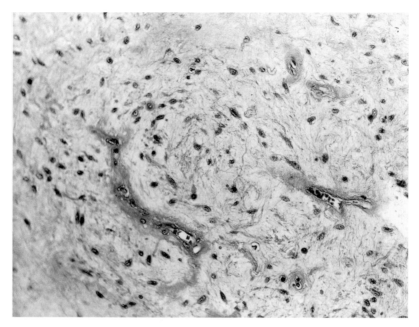

Fig. 191. *Aggressive angiomyxoma,* vulva. Myxoid tissue containing blood vessels with slightly thickened walls

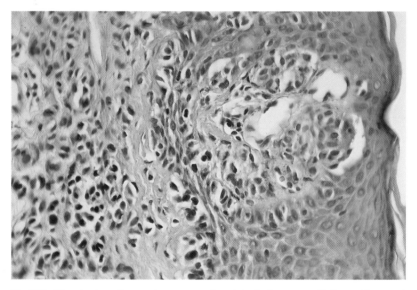

Fig. 192. *Dysplastic melanocytic naevus,* vulva. Atypical naevus cells in papillary and reticular dermis

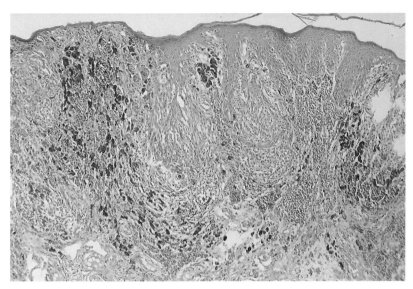

Fig. 193. *Malignant melanoma*, vulva. Pigmented and nonpigmented spindle cells diffusely replacing upper dermis

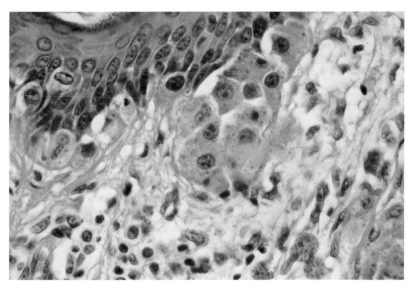

Fig. 194. *Malignant melanoma,* vulva. Large rounded cells with central nuclei and prominent nucleoli and with pigmented, abundant cytoplasm at junction of epidermis and dermis

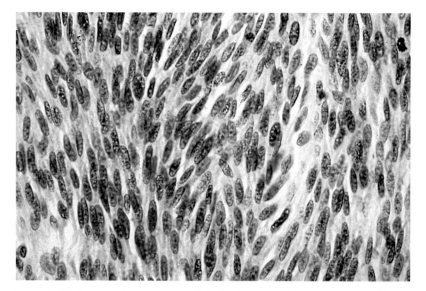

Fig. 195. *Malignant melanoma,* vulva. Spindle-shaped nuclei creating a resemblance to spindle cell sarcoma

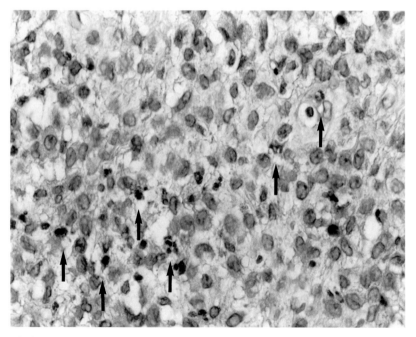

Fig. 196. *Langerhans cell histiocytosis,* vulva. Diffuse proliferation of histiocytes with a few eosinophils *(arrows)*

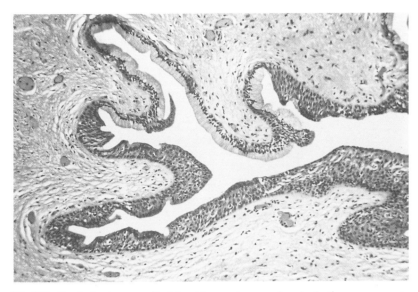

Fig. 197. *Bartholin duct cyst.* Cyst lined by mucinous and metaplastic squamous epithelium

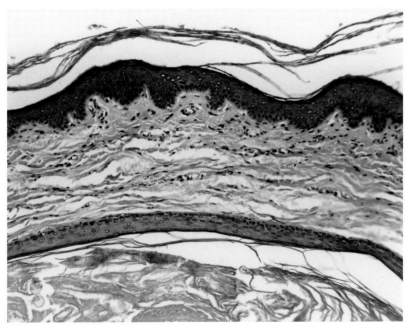

Fig. 198. *Epidermal cyst.* Cyst filled with keratin and lined by thin layer of squamous epithelium

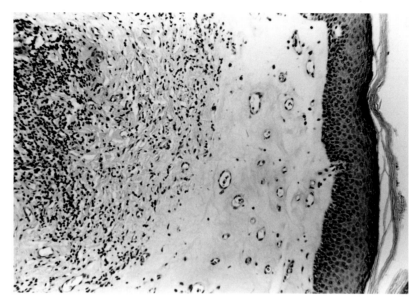

Fig. 199. *Lichen sclerosus,* vulva. Loss of rete ridges, homogeneous, parvicellular subepithelial layer and deep layer containing numerous round cells

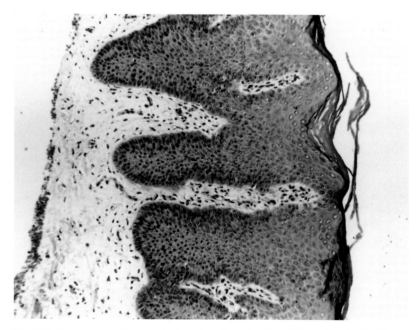

Fig. 200. *Squamous cell hyperplasia,* vulva. Acanthosis and hyperkeratosis without atypia and without features of specific forms of dermatosis or dermatitis

Subject Index